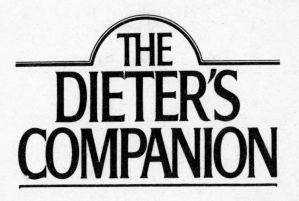

THE
DIETER'S
COMPANION

Other Avon Books by
Judy Moscovitz

THE RICE DIET REPORT

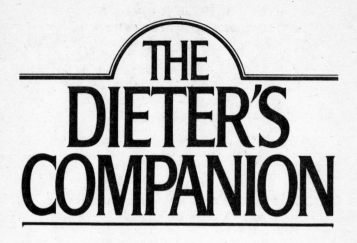

THE DIETER'S COMPANION

JUDY MOSCOVITZ

AVON BOOKS ◆ NEW YORK

For Irving Silver,
with gratitude for your kind
heart and unfailing support

THE DIETER'S COMPANION is an original publication of Avon Books. This work has never before appeared in book form.

AVON BOOKS
A division of
The Hearst Corporation
105 Madison Avenue
New York, New York 10016

First Avon Books Trade Printing: March 1989

AVON TRADEMARK REG. U.S. PAT. OFF. AND IN OTHER COUNTRIES, MARCA REGISTRADA, HECHO EN U.S.A.

Printed in the U.S.A.

OPM 10 9 8 7 6 5 4 3 2 1

SPECIAL ACKNOWLEDGMENT

If credit were to be given where credit is due, many of the ideas expressed in this book would be prefaced by the words "As Dr. Kempner says . . . "

As this would obviously be most tedious for the reader, I will say it just once:

I am forever indebted to Dr. Walter Kempner of Duke University for the insights and support he has given me over the years. I hope I have done justice to his vision and his work.

ACKNOWLEDGMENTS

First of all, for my mother, Bess Moscovitz, with gratitude for a lifetime of love and an example I can only aspire to.

For my sister, Irma Berlin, and her children, Amy, Andy and Richard, and for my cousin, Julia Saul.

For my friends, who have truly loved me through thick and thin: Melinda Joy Katzman, Sandra "Pappy" Steinberg, Bryan Knight, Randy Norris, Barbara Northrup, Lilah Poncé, Carol Prives, Judy Altman, Liz Oglesby, Johanne Johnson, Nancy Yoos, Marge Southern, Rose and David Ronne, Evelyn Lazar, Sheree Letovsky and Naomi Schimel.

For the medical professionals whose skill and support made all the difference in the world: Dr. Mercedes Gaffron, Dr. Barbara Newborg, Dr. Robert Rosati, Norma Neal, Sister Celeste, Bob Horn, and the entire staff at the Rice House; Dr. David Wood, Dr. Nathan Wisebord, Dr. Lawrence K. Thompson III and his staff, particularly Paul S. Toth and Karen Bryant, and Dr. Brian Ticoll of Montreal.

To the other professionals who do so well the things I cannot do: my editor, Susanne Jaffe; my agent, Mort Janklow, and his colleagues, Anne Sibbald, Maria Gallacher and Cynthia Cannell; Monroe Gardner in Raleigh and Chris Pappas in New York.

And one special word of thanks to my beloved dog, my Goldie.

TABLE OF CONTENTS

INTRODUCTION

A Letter to My Readers

𝔇ear Fellow Dieter,

In 1982, I lost 140 pounds. Unquestionably, it was the hardest thing I have ever done.

The fact that losing weight is so difficult is attested to by the reality that so few do it, despite the plethora of information and a nationwide focus on weight that is virtually an obsession.

At any given time, sixty-five million Americans are dieting. That includes nearly half of all adult women and a quarter of all adult men. A total of ten billion dollars a year is spent on various methods of losing weight. Most of these attempts at weight loss are justified: according to *Prevention* magazine, less than a quarter of American adults are at the recommended weight for their age, sex and height.

Yet where has all this expense and effort gotten us? Despite the fitness craze, the average American is six pounds heavier today than twenty years ago. Nothing that we try seems to work. The more conservative methods, like counting calories, have not met with noticeable success. Appetite suppressants have not been found to be useful; psychological intervention has rarely helped.

2

This has led to a proliferation of more drastic approaches—wiring jaws, intestinal bypasses, stomach-stapling, etc. Most of these procedures have unpleasant and possibly fatal side effects, and withal, their results cannot be said to be impressive.

Nor have traditional diet books been of much help. The best (or the most bizarre) rush to the top of the best-seller list, only to be knocked off a few months later by the latest entry in the diet sweepstakes. Though these books sell in the millions, there is little evidence that they help. No one seems to lose very much weight; what little is lost is usually put right back on. If anything, the population seems to be getting more and more out of shape.

Although many of these diets unquestionably lack value, I do not think that the main fault lies with the diets themselves. The problem is that a diet—even a good one—is simply not enough. Successful weight loss must go beyond diet—it must be seen as a learning experience. Unfortunately, most people do not stick with a diet long enough to learn what they need to know.

Nor has there been anywhere to look for this information. To the best of my knowledge, there is no published treatment of the nondiet issues that can affect one's weight, no compendium of practical advice that goes beyond dietary guidelines.

This book is intended to fill that gap. I want to tell you the things I wish I had known twenty years ago—the helpful information that can make diet misery a thing of the past.

3

The topics I will be discussing are relevant to those with any amount of weight to lose, from the minimally overweight to the obese.

Weight control is an area filled with theory, much of it contradictory. Despite the glut of nutrition information, no two experts seem to agree. Well, I have been in the trenches with this issue, and I believe my opinion is as valid as most. To be perfectly honest, I think I understand it better than most, because, after all, I have lived it, not just studied about it in books. All of us with weight problems must walk the same road. I presume to give advice because I am six years farther along this path.

I will try to be completely honest about what I believe to be true, but I feel obliged to tell you that every now and then, something I say is bound to be wrong. After all, with so many opinions about so many topics, I'm bound to miss the boat every once in a while!

Nonetheless, I hope you'll hear me out, because I believe I can help you get from where you are to where you want to be. It's sort of like the old man who turns one hundred and attracts dozens of reporters asking him the secret of his long life. The presumption is, "Hey, this guy actually *did* it. He must know something. Maybe there's something I can learn."

Like his advice, mine comes from actual experience. I've been fat. I lost weight (quickly, too!), and I've kept it off for six years. To me it seems reasonable that I might know something that can be of help.

And I really *do* want to help, if I possibly can, because I know what a difference losing weight will make in your life. Losing weight doesn't just get you thin; it prevents suffering, both emotional and physical. To be thin is to be youthful and vital, to feel alive with energy and health. To be overweight, even a little, is to deprive yourself of much of what life has to offer.

Yes, I *am* a fanatic on the subject of weight, and I want to make you a fanatic, too. Not obsessed (which is boring and stressful), but committed to being your best—which is what proper eating is really all about.

Losing weight is undoubtedly hard, but

it is worth it, because it affects virtually every aspect of your life. It affects your career and your relationships; it affects your health, your mood and your self-esteem.

Nobody likes to be fat, nobody wants to be fat—yet plenty are. But change is possible, good things are possible; the way you are now is not the way you have to be. To lose weight is to become a different person, because the external change is inevitably matched by an internal transformation. To change your eating habits is to change your life—and, I promise you, for the better.

If you're overweight, my heart goes out to you, and I hope this book will be of help.

5

Love,

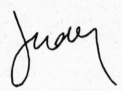

SELF-CONCEPT AND
THE "ME" BOOK

How Do Others Really See You?

Most of us are concerned with how we are seen by others; too often we're convinced that others see us in a negative light. More often than not, this is a *distortion*, not a *reflection*, of reality. To the extent that others think of us at all, they are usually neutral or positive in judgment.

Generally speaking, others see us in two ways: as a physical being and as the kind of person we are. And usually, others' perceptions are more accurate than our own. Most of us are all too aware of our actual or perceived shortcomings. We tend to be critical of ourselves; we are our own worst judge.

Our lack of clear vision about ourselves leads to low self-esteem. Obviously you can't be self-confident if you think you're a miserable failure.

Well, there's a solution to this, a way of learning to see ourselves more accurately. I suggest that you start keeping a "Me" book, an ongoing written record of whatever feedback about yourself you receive. In the course of your daily life, people frequently offer comments on how they perceive you. Seeing those accumulate in print can provide you with a pretty clear picture of how you come across. Just jot the words down verbatim in any notebook.

8

A "Me" book can be a useful tool for anyone, but it is particularly helpful for those who are losing weight. In some ways, losing weight means becoming a different person; for many, it involves a truly radical change. You may find yourself becoming something of a stranger to yourself. Who *is* this new person? How do others see and feel about you?

When I first lost weight, I experienced a degree of understandable uncertainty about who I really was, and at that time I began keeping a "Me" book of my own. I was hungry for whatever knowledge I could acquire about this new person I saw in the mirror, and I began jotting down everything people said to me about myself. In short order, I had acquired invaluable information, and I soon began to develop and internalize a much clearer picture of my-self.

Those who undertake a "Me" book are likely to find that certain comments keep recurring, and they thus can be pretty sure that that is, indeed, how they are viewed. If people use the same words about you over and over, you have to conclude that that *must* be who you are, how you come across.

To give you an example, one of the new self-definitions I heard was the word "pe-tite." What, *me* petite??!! You've got to be kidding! Yet many people used that word to describe me (or variations of it, like "tiny," or "no bigger than a minute"). Impossible as it seemed, I concluded that it must be true! After a while, I genuinely and inter-nally *knew* that I was, indeed, small. But it was so alien to my lifelong self-concept that if I hadn't been absorbing what others were perceiving, I would have had the greatest difficulty believing it was so.

9

Even those not involved in weight loss can benefit from writing down feedback of all kinds that they hear about themselves. We often think that people have opinions about us that are, in fact, very far from the truth. And what we *think* they think is usually much more negative than their ac-tual assessment. Almost invariably we find that we are evaluated more highly than we expected. This new knowledge results in an improved perception of self. Frankly, it's a whole lot easier to think you're wonderful when others tell you how wonderful *they* think you are!

Naturally, you have to write down negative feedback as well. A "Me" book is not intended to be one of those pop psych, feel-good endeavors, but an accurate reflection of how others see you, warts and all. Regard it as information gathering, an attempt to form a genuine picture of yourself as seen by others.

10

It is also a source of self-transformation, in that it can help you zero in on what needs work. You will find it helpful to look back on over the years, to see how you have changed and grown.

Of course, the flip side of this is that you should tell others how you see and feel about them so that they, too, can incorporate more accurate ideas into their self-perception. In particular, never hesitate to give a compliment, even to a total stranger. If you *think* something nice, say it out loud—why ever not? How can it hurt to make someone feel good?

It helped me enormously to compile and study my "Me" book, and I think you will find it an eye-opener (and a lot of fun!), too.

DOES LOSING WEIGHT CHANGE YOUR LIFE?

The pain of being overweight may not lead to weight loss, but it sure does lead to dreams. Fantasies of what your life *could* be like, if only you were thin.

Most diet books exhort you to lose weight, but caution you not to expect your life to change just because you do. My reaction to that is always, "Are you kidding?" NOTHING will change your life as totally as learning to eat properly and getting to an ideal weight. There is no aspect of your life that will remain unaffected by this one change.

To the extent that you are overweight, to that extent the real you never even gets a chance to live. Obesity is a very self-absorbed, inward way of living, an anti-life stance, nothing less than a living death. If you are spending a good deal of time focusing on food, weight and diets, it doesn't really matter if you have ten or a hundred pounds to lose. The real loss is of time, the precious moments of your life.

I was always so absorbed in the subject of my weight that I sometimes wondered what would fill the hours if I got thin and was no longer obsessed. I now have my answer. *Life* rushes in to fill the gap. Since nature abhors a vacuum, you may be sure that all kinds of wondrous things will fill the void once thoughts of food are mercifully removed.

12

Being thin is not as good as you are hoping. It is infinitely better. But it is not the most important thing; in truth, it is only a fringe benefit. True, most of the time it is vanity that moves us to diet—the desire to look good, wear small-sized clothes and strut our stuff. But you can be thin while eating junk and still remain far from your best. The real transformation comes from giving your body the exact foods it needs. Only then can you be not only thin but at your peak.

What changes can you expect from feeding your body properly? Nothing less than a complete transformation in your life. Not only will you look better, you will feel healthy, wonderful and strong. You will be energetic and alert instead of tired and lethargic. People will tell you you look radiant; you'll have vitality to spare.

One important difference will be your ability to handle stress. When your eating is out of control, life's problems seem overwhelming. When you are eating properly, you somehow always feel able to cope.

You will be more positive and optimistic, more loving to the people in your life. You will look forward to every day and at last know true peace of mind.

Though obviously it encompasses appearance, weight loss is more significantly an issue of power. You empower yourself when you feed your body the foods it was meant to eat, just as you reduce your power immeasurably when you put bad foods in your mouth. I do not mean power over others (although you will certainly have more power in your relationships and on the job), but rather a power felt internally, a feeling of exultance, a surge of life.

13

The more successful you are in this endeavor, the more self-confidence you will gain. With calmness, peace and inner strength, *you will stop settling for less.*

These changes, this progress, are virtually inevitable. This new life *must* come to you, this new person who CAN DO. Losing weight is a difficult undertaking, requiring curiosity, passion and faith. To lose weight—to choose consistently to eat in a way that's to your advantage—is to prove that you are special. It's not just choosing a new way of living. In a profound sense, it's choosing *life.*

I cannot guarantee that eating properly and losing weight will help you attain all your dreams, but I *can* promise that you will be better equipped to handle *whatever* the future holds.

DOES WHAT DIET
YOU FOLLOW
MAKE ANY DIFFERENCE?

In my dieting days, I tried virtually every diet that came down the pike. I did Scarsdale, Atkins, Stillman, the Beverly Hills diet, the grapefruit diet and the dozen or so different diets purporting to come from The Mayo Clinic.

I never thought of a diet as anything but a means of getting thin. Since then, however, I have learned that a diet must be much more. The ideal diet should not only help you lose weight, it should also make you healthier and more energetic, eliminate the need for most medications, and help prevent degenerative diseases over the long term.

Most critically, in order to be worth anything at all, a diet must teach you how to eat for life so that your weight loss will be permanent.

Dieting is a field rife with contradictions, misinformation and downright ignorance. Yesterday's dogma is today's old wives' tale—which makes you wonder which of today's beliefs will be discredited tomorrow.

Nonetheless, there is a great deal of research and evidence pointing in one clear direction: the best diets are those that are low in sodium, sugar and fat, moderate in protein (be it from animal or vegetable sources) and high in fiber and complex carbohydrates. Any good diet is bound to come down to these basic truths. That's simply the way man was intended by nature to eat. The fact is that the human body is a mechanism, no different from any other. Certain foods will cause the body to thrive; other foods will cause it to degenerate. The diet one selects must take more into consideration than losing weight.

A diet based on the above principles will not only help you lose weight but can be regarded as preventive medicine. Not only does such a diet pay off in long-term results, it will also permit you to lose weight very quickly, which I believe is to your benefit. This brings us to one of the questions I hear most often:

IS IT BETTER TO LOSE WEIGHT QUICKLY OR SLOWLY?

Like you, for years I have heard that it is better to lose weight slowly, because that makes it likelier that you'll keep it off. This statement has been repeated so often, people accept it without question. I don't agree. If anything, I think a good case could be made that if you're overweight, the quicker you get it off, the better.

I believe you might as well pick a quick weight-loss diet instead of a slow one, as long as the diet you choose is healthy in nature. A quick weight-loss diet is no harder than one that permits you more food. Deprivation is deprivation, and no sane diet is going to permit you to eat the sweets and junk you crave. Moreover, when you see you're losing quickly, you're more motivated to see it through.

Sometimes you hear people say that rapid weight loss is "only water," but where's the problem in that? After all, our bodies are composed of 70 percent water, so inevitably water will represent a major part of any loss on any diet. The fact remains that when you lose ten pounds of *anything*, you weigh ten pounds less and you look ten pounds thinner. Your clothes fit ten pounds better and you have that much less to lose.

MAKING THE CHANGE

A diet of plain, natural food is not hard to accommodate. There is much *less* to be done. Yes, it demands a radical change, but modest alterations will lead to only modest improvements, and why should you settle for being anything but your best?

Realize that it will take time to fully incorporate this new way of eating into your life. You have to totally undo the eating habits of a lifetime, as well as the acquired physical distortions of taste. Stick to it, though, and you will gain dominion instead of pounds. Indeed, with time, you will not even want those foods that are now calling to you and making you miserable. The vast majority of the foods I used to "love" I now wouldn't touch, even if they had absolutely no calories in them. I still love food, but I have changed the focus of that love. This makes it (almost!) easy for me to stay thin.

Eating healthily gives you life. Eating junk simply satisfies an impulse. You can learn to love plain food every bit as much as you love the foods you are presently eating, and without having to pay any short- or long-term price. It is only a question of willingness—willingness, effort and time. It isn't easy, but it's worth it, because the alternative is fighting this same battle all your life.

Frankly, it's not enough to want to be

thin. *Everyone* wants to be thin. You have to be willing to pay the price. You have to be willing to give up most of the destructive eating you do. Eliminate the unhealthy foods completely if you can, but be ready to settle for improvement instead of a cure.

This way of eating is not what you are used to—but you can *get* used to it if you so choose. Health and good looks taste much better than gourmet fare.

Changing your eating habits is undeniably hard, but if you are willing to do it, you will quite literally transform your life. Giving up "normal" eating may be difficult, but it is a heck of a lot easier than going through life fat.

BEATING THE SCALE
BLUES

*Don't Let the Numbers
Get You Down*

From my very earliest years the scale has had power over my emotions.

I can still remember the twice-yearly weigh-ins in elementary school, when one nurse would weigh us, then call our weight across the room to a second nurse, who would record it on our charts. This let the whole class know how much I weighed, which led to comments like "Gee, you weigh more than my mother!" or "Boy, you sure are fat." I hated weigh-in days, and I still remember them with mortification.

The scale still remains a power to be reckoned with, but there *are* ways of diminishing the effect it can have. I consider this crucial for peace of mind.

I am profoundly troubled by the amount of time, energy, effort and emotion we—particularly women—put into the issues of food, diet and weight. We are so bombarded with images of thinness that it is virtually impossible to be satisfied with our bodies, no matter how nice they may be. Research indicates that even women who are *underweight* are anxious about their bodies and constantly dieting.

22

I believe in getting thin. More importantly, I believe in eating right. But matters of diet and weight have become an unhealthy obsession in this country, with some women taking laxatives or diuretics, or throwing up to maintain their weight.

Anxiety over weight and body shape is affecting the lives of a sizable (no pun intended) segment of the population. Poor body image is the rule, rather than the exception, regardless of what the reality of a person's appearance is.

A lot of this misery focuses on the number we see each morning on the scale. We are much too tied in to numbers, when what we should be worrying about is what we are putting into our mouths. Eat properly and don't worry—the scale will take care of itself. After all, if obsessing were productive, we'd all be reed-thin by now!

Remember that the number on the scale is essentially meaningless. It vacillates all the time, for many reasons—or for no reason at all. Who among us has not had the experience of dieting seriously, only to see no difference on the scale? Who has not occasionally overeaten, yet still shown a loss? Certainly there's a connection between what you eat and whether you lose or gain, but that connection is not necessarily manifested immediately.

We like to believe that there are particular actions we can take that will be followed by specific results. For example, if we diet on Tuesday, we must necessarily show a loss on Wednesday. Unfortunately, that ain't necessarily so. It is even possible to diet conscientiously, yet show a gain! Our bodies are subject to random fluctuations, no matter how we eat on any individual day. This is normal, natural and nothing to worry about. All that's important is to hang in.

23

Of course, hanging in can be hard when we don't see the loss we're anticipating. Yet no matter how much we lose, we feel it is never enough. Whatever the scale shows, we are vaguely disappointed. Dieters are impatient people. They not only want results, they want results *now*. (My favorite story concerns the dieter who complained to me one day that she wasn't losing fast enough. I told her, "The trouble with you is that you want to be thin by tomorrow." "Why tomorrow?" she asked. "Is today booked?")

Our weight loss tends to get mixed up with our sense of what's "fair." It somehow isn't "fair" that we didn't lose, or didn't lose enough, after a good diet day. Or perhaps it's not "fair" that a friend ate more than we did, yet lost weight, while we gained. We blame the diet, and want to quit. Alas, fairness has nothing to do with it; reality often defies the way we think things should be. We must learn to deal patiently and reasonably with reality, because our sense of injustice won't affect our weight one whit.

24

Discouragement may be understandable, but it is counterproductive. What's important is to remember that physiological laws apply: eating wisely—*consistently*—will lead to eventual success. Stick to it over the long haul, and the weight will come off. This is as unalterable a fact as "two plus two equals four."

To avoid being traumatized by the scale, some dieters prefer to skip weighing themselves altogether. I am strongly against this, as it most often leads to self-deception and weight gain. I recall the friend who told me in all seriousness that she gained twenty pounds because she installed wall-to-wall carpeting in her house. Seems that the carpet distorted her scale's readout, so she had to stop weighing herself. When I asked if her clothes didn't get tight, she said that she thought they had all shrunk in the wash. It is, alas, all too easy to tell ourselves stories when we're not forced to face facts.

I believe you should weigh yourself once

daily, preferably first thing in the morning, before getting dressed. And I mean *every* day, *especially* if you've cheated. That is the very worst time to avoid the scale. How can you accomplish anything if you're not even dealing with reality? It's important to learn to handle both failure and success. Coping with consequences is an important aspect of maturity, and the development of maturity is a large part of what weight loss is all about.

25

Do not, however, weigh yourself more than once a day. I have been known to weigh myself before and after going to the bathroom, before and after getting a haircut and even before and after biting off my nails. This is nutsy behavior, and neither you nor I should be doing it. *Do* weigh yourself, but keep it within reasonable bounds. By all means, take your diet seriously, but don't allow the number on the scale to rule or ruin your life.

Regard weighing yourself as simply a learning experience, a chance to evaluate your progress. However, do not focus on attaining any particular number. To our minds, our "ideal weight" represents some final form of victory, some ultimate success. This magical thinking suggests that if we only weighed our ideal weight, our lives would be okay.

A much more valid goal is the accumulation of good diet days. Remember that a "good diet day" can be anything from one where you ate only 700 calories to one where you ate less than usual at an all-you-can-eat buffet. It is relative, not absolute, and it leads, at last, to peace of mind.

KEEPING WEIGHT OFF
IS *NOT*
HARDER THAN LOSING IT

The popular theory is that, hard as it is to take weight off, it is even harder to keep it off once you've lost it. I think this is ridiculous. It is *much* easier to keep weight off once you're thin.

In my opinion, this is an old wives' tale, and a destructive one to boot. It' discourages people from dieting even before they begin. "What, hard as it is to lose weight, it's going to be even harder once I'm thin??!!" Understandably, a dieter might decide to throw in the towel.

This chapter explores the different factors that influence whether or not you're likely to keep off the weight you lose. Let's take a look at the issues involved.

LOSING WITH THE RIGHT DIET

If you lose weight with an unbalanced fad diet, the odds of your keeping it off will be slim. After all, what have you learned that will help you over the long term?

I believe that a well-planned, healthy diet will give you all the tools on the way down that you will need to know once you have arrived. In other words, there should be no real difference between your weight-loss diet and your maintenance diet. Some extra foods will be added, and you'll increase the quantity of food you're allowed, but that's about it.

28

A good, well-constructed diet doesn't get harder, it gets easier over time. You get used to making the right choices, used to feeling light, feeling good. You become less interested in food. The times you overeat are now the *bad* times, not the "treats." You simply feel so much better when you feed your body right.

A diet must be regarded as a learning experience. It is not some ridiculous break in your normal routine during which you eat nothing but lettuce leaves or cottage cheese. It is the initial phase of what must be a lifelong routine. It's a time to pay your dues, retrain your body and learn what you need to know.

You may be tempted to try all the fad diets that come out, but what's the good of a diet if it doesn't teach you anything? So what if it managed to crash some weight off? You can't fad-diet forever, nor can you go back to the way you ate before. Yet your diet will have taught you no alternate eating behaviors. Only a well-balanced, healthy diet will do this.

The weight-loss part of your diet must lead *naturally* into maintenance. Desperate short-term measures will not do.

GETTING GENUINELY THIN

29

I know, the statistics are grim. Only two to three percent of those who lose weight keep it off. Ninety percent of those who lose gain it back within a year.

But what do these statistics really mean?

The implication is that people get thin, then regain their weight. What really happens is that most people lose some weight (as opposed to *getting thin*), then put that lost weight back on. In other words, a man who has to lose thirty pounds stays on a diet long enough to take off ten, then stops dieting. Naturally, he easily puts those ten pounds back on. He hasn't stuck with the diet long enough to learn what he needs to know. He is only minimally removed from his original overweight self. He may have lost weight, but what he has done is essentially meaningless.

This kind of partial weight loss can be compared to the student who completes only three years of medical school, then quits. Unless he completes his degree, of what use to him are those three years? They are not "better than nothing"—they are a senseless waste of time. Like him, unless you go all the way, you have achieved nothing you can use. It is not enough to get *thinner*. You must get actually *thin*.

30

I would wager that the statistics for permanent weight loss are significantly higher for those who go all the way to goal. It is much easier to keep weight off when you are feeling and looking good. The payoffs help keep you honest. Moreover, you will have taken the time to learn what you need to know.

There is little long-term advantage in going from fat to less fat. The only real transformation comes in going from fat to thin.

DISTANCING YOURSELF FROM AN INAPPROPRIATE LOVE OF FOOD

It is much easier to keep away from destructive foods if you learn not to love them so much. This is a question of changing your tastes, and it is not particularly difficult if you are willing to move in this direction. The person who manages to lose weight while retaining a preference for unhealthy foods is very unlikely to stay slim. If you aim at learning to prefer fruits, grains, and vegetables, your chances for long-term success are greatly enhanced.

This does not mean never eating "bad"

foods again—I wouldn't dream of asking of you the impossible. But it does mean that those foods can't play a regular part in your life.

If you keep loving those foods that will harm you, you are always engaged in a struggle with yourself. Sometimes you'll win, but all too often, food will be the victor. And even if you win, what a strain on yourself! I am tired of living in hand-to-hand combat with food; I am tired of fighting this particular battle. I would just as soon be more indifferent to food. It makes staying thin so much easier.

31

Anyone can occasionally go off a diet and remain thin, but no one can go back full-time to his or her old ways of eating. This means a commitment to eating by new rules. Yes, you should eat what you truly enjoy, but the trick is to learn to enjoy foods that are good for you. This is not at all difficult if you are *willing* to make the change.

The fact is that overindulgence is usually not an agreeable experience. The first few bites are sublime; then it's downhill all the way. I have found it helpful to ask myself from time to time, "Do I want this? Do I like it? Am I enjoying it? Would I buy (or make) it again?" If the answer to any of these questions is no, then why should I continue eating it? Makes no sense to me.

We have a distorted idea of a "treat." We think of treats as sweet or heavily sauced foods that are bad for us. Work at learning to prefer less destructive alternatives. I have found that dried figs, dates and raisins can satisfy my sweet tooth. (Medjool dates are as creamy and sweet as chocolate.) A small handful of unsalted nuts provides the crunch offered by cookies. Frozen pureed fruits substitute well for ice cream.

Some of those alternatives are relatively high in calories, but I still regard them as a superior choice. They're intrinsically healthy, and they don't arouse cravings for more. Best of all, when I eat them, I feel neither worried nor guilty.

32

One way to wean yourself from destructive preferences is to keep away from eating them for as long as you can. Eat ice cream on Monday, and on Tuesday it will tempt you again. Don't eat it for a couple of weeks, and it will be a lot less tempting. The longer you put off eating bad foods, the greater your chances of losing interest in them completely.

I have now reached the point where I *prefer* to eat plain food. Occasionally, I still want some of the old-time junk, but over time, these desires have become increasingly infrequent. And after a bout with the baddies, I am always glad to get back on track. Healthy food is so delicious that a good diet day and a good eating day have become synonymous.

People sometimes ask me if I still "treat" myself, and I know they mean do I still eat junk food and sweets. Indeed I do, but the days when I indulge in those foods are far from "treats"; they are the *bad* days. Eating unhealthily does not make me feel either better or happier—on the contrary. The *real* treats are the days I manage to limit myself to healthy foods.

ACKNOWLEDGING THE CONTINUED EXISTENCE OF A FOOD PROBLEM

Listen to some of those ads for weight-loss clinics, and you'll hear some happy client announce, "I lost weight by doing such and such, and I'm never going to put it back on again."

So far I've kept my weight off for six years, and I feel increasingly confident, but I would *never* say I'll never put it on again. I figure when they pack me away into my final resting place, I'll know whether or not I made it. Until then, I keep soberly aware that I have to contend with an eating problem.

People don't like to hear that after they've lost weight they will still have problems with food, but unfortunately, that's the reality. There is no permanent solution, no trouble-free existence. I think it is crucial that you remember this, because if you don't keep a vigilant awareness, you will be in trouble soon. Your problems with weight may have ended, but your problems with food and eating remain. To believe anything else is to buy into wishful thinking.

KEEPING ON TOP OF YOUR WEIGHT

For obvious reasons, it is crucial to nip any weight gain in the bud.

No need to worry as long as you're within your acceptable range (see "Is the American Body Ideal Too Thin?"), but if you're even one pound over, you should immediately cut down. All you need at that point is one good diet day.

34

Be sure to weigh yourself daily so you'll know where you stand.

BEING ASSERTIVE

To stay thin requires taking responsibility for making it happen. You must be willing to speak up in restaurants and when being entertained. This is a food-oriented society, and temptations and pressures abound. If you don't make your diet a priority, you won't stand much of a chance. You must be committed to getting your needs met in almost every circumstance.

If being exacting makes you uncomfortable, ask yourself what you would do if you were sick. If you had diabetes or heart disease, you know you'd insist on getting what you need. *Your* condition is every bit as serious, and it is critical that you treat it as such. Do what is necessary to take care of yourself.

GETTING INVOLVED WITH LIFE

Though I believe overeating is a physiological disorder, I know there is an emotional component as well. I do not see it as a psychological problem, but rather as a result of being lonely and bored. The antidote, as I see it, is to get involved with life.

Developing your natural curiosity will help you control your weight. Keep busy, keep active, look for ways in which you can contribute. Your problems with eating don't stem from hunger, but from concentrated focusing on food. Shift your thinking to another arena—this will help immeasurably in keeping off weight.

35

TAKING CARE OF YOURSELF

After I had lost about a hundred pounds, one of the men at the Rice House took me aside and made some suggestions. His point was that getting thin wasn't enough —I should also start wearing makeup, trade my glasses for contacts and buy myself some new clothes. I was outraged. Was nothing I did enough???

But he was right. When you look good in every way, you feel terrific, interesting things happen to you more often and it becomes easier to stay thin. Good grooming pays off, both short- and long-term.

MOVING ON

Losing weight is not just a physical change. Properly implemented, it is a learning process. You change not just externally, but internally, psychologically, as well.

36

For many of us, all we know is dieting or cheating. We're either on a diet or off; we're either gaining weight or losing it. Once we're thin, it can be hard to turn this central focus into a nonissue. There can be anxiety attached to letting the obsession with dieting go. Still, there is an appropriate time to put this issue into perspective.

You will never forget about it completely, nor would that be a wise thing to do. But there *does* come a time to put it aside and wipe the blackboard clean. To continue obsessing about weight long after the job has been done is unhealthy. It can keep you as anxious and unhappy as when you were actually overweight.

You must keep the *learning* of the past, but leave the negative aspects behind you. You've done what you undertook to do. Now stay aware, but get on with your life.

GETTING BACK ON TRACK

THE PERFECT DIET VS. REALITY

I happen to know all about getting back on a diet, because I'm forever falling off one. I may no longer have a *weight* problem, but my *food* problem is far from gone. I still binge, I still eat junk food and I still occasionally gain weight—but I sure manage my food problem better than I ever did before.

And that's really all one can hope for. Seeing a diet through to goal does not mean being a perfect dieter. Indeed, unless you have only a few pounds to lose, it is completely unreasonable for you to think you will start a diet and never once stray. After all, you are, by definition, a person with a food problem, and that is not going to disappear just because you have "decided" to go on a diet. A diet means struggle and intermittent failure, and the successful dieter is the one who can incorporate the occasional binge into his or her life.

Please understand, I am in no way recommending that you cheat on your diet. I am only saying that the odds are that you will. Probably again and again—and what's the problem with that?

Most dieters get thrown when they cheat —they regard it as the end of the diet. Which is why most people run from diet to diet, equating success with perfection and failure with even the smallest lapse.

What's one thing got to do with another? A lapse is just a lapse, a short detour along the road. It may be undesirable, and I know it can be upsetting, but it doesn't essentially *matter*. It means absolutely nothing in terms of your eventual success.

The problem, you see, isn't that you've broken the diet. The problem is that you don't get right back on. No error is significant unless you refuse to correct it, and a binge nipped in the bud is just an opportunity to learn.

You must, of course, make every effort to fight off your desire to eat, but it's also important to realize that sometimes you'll lose this fight. This is reality. And since you probably can't ever completely eradicate this behavior, you have no alternative but to adapt and learn to live with it.

Just like the occasional fight doesn't

mean that you've picked the wrong man and this is the end of the marriage, the occasional lapse or binge doesn't mean you've picked the wrong diet or that the diet is at an end. In both of these cases, you must absorb the difficult time, hopefully learn from it, and go on from there. Diets and marriages require long-term commitment and the decision to see it through, be it good times or bad. And you must expect both—they're part of the terrain.

Nor is there any call for self-recrimination and guilt. You're a person with a food problem, and you're struggling with it as best you can. Learn to correct yourself without condemning yourself. After all, if you can't adjust to the occasional failure, how can you ever hope to succeed? If nothing short of the perfect diet is acceptable, you'll likely be overweight for life. Accept your human frailty; just try to improve. Forget about perfection—*progress* is good enough for now.

ONE GOOD DAY

All right, you've cheated, you've accepted it, now it's time to get back on track. Only you're afraid you can't do it, and you're miserable about the pounds you've put back on.

If you're like most of us, at this point you start thinking punitively. You decide to cut down even more—maybe even fast—to quickly get those pounds off. Big mistake

—don't do it. When you're having a rough time with a diet, that's the very worst time to consider making it even more stringent.

Forget the number on the scale. All you need is *one good day.* One good day may not take off what you've put on, but that is irrelevant. It will get your head back in a good place, make you once again feel calm and in control.

40

I cannot overemphasize the importance of this perspective. Nice as it would be, at this point you don't need to be thin. You don't even need to be rid of the weight you've gained. One good day will rout despondency; your feelings of hopelessness and fear will be gone. You will once again believe that this is something you can do. In just one day of healthy, appropriate eating, the tension caused by your out-of-control episode will disappear and you'll feel calm, confident and optimistic once again.

Make no mistake, it will require a great deal of effort to achieve that one good day. It's hard to get back on a diet after even the slightest lapse, and the longer you've been off the diet, the harder it will be to return.

Since overeating engages you on physical, mental and emotional levels, it must be fought on those three levels as well. Breaking a binge's grip on you requires substituting something other than food in your thoughts, feelings and actions.

I can suggest a few of the techniques that have helped me get back on track

when I've fallen off. It is a case of fighting
fire with fire. Since overeating is part of an
obsessive pattern, I try to replace my destructive obsessiveness with productive
obsessiveness. I keep busy by doing one or
more of the following:

ACTIONS

Well, this one won't make me popular,
but I have found that the best thing to do
instead of reaching for food is housework.
Nothing you absolutely hate, of course, like
scrubbing floors or washing windows, but
easy kinds of busywork that make the
place shine. Clean counters, iron, dust, go
through closets or drawers, attend to some
sewing—that kind of thing. This not only
keeps you busy, it also provides some physical activity and pays off by improving your
environment. Moreover, it makes you feel
good about yourself and dispels some of
those negative thoughts you've been having.

41

THOUGHTS

To occupy my mind when trying to get
back on a diet, I frequently start what I call
a Productivity Journal. This is any old
notebook in which I jot down in detail the
productive things I do in any one-hour period, from the time I wake up until I go to
sleep at night. This is particularly helpful

when you are ravaged by a longing for food; it keeps you busy and out of the supermarket.

In a sense, what we need during tough times is to have our hand held, and an hourly check-in chart serves as that always-present helping hand. Carry your notebook with you wherever you go, and mark in each entry as soon as you have completed the activity.

42

Obviously, this is not an important record, and I never keep it or reread it, but it does somehow help me get through difficult days. I am the first to agree that this is very obsessive behavior, but hey, we already know you're obsessive, no? Better *directed* obsessiveness than out-of-control obsessiveness.

I recommend that you do this for a day or two, until you feel safely back on course. If you've been out of control for several days or more, I suggest you do it for at least four days, because it can take that long to get over the withdrawal symptoms from addictive foods.

Yes, it is busywork, but it is an excellent substitute for eating, and best of all, it *works*.

A typical day's entry might look something like this:

7–8 a.m.	Get up. Brush teeth. Put on makeup.
8–9 a.m.	Get dressed. Call Mother. Call to have cable TV installed. Make dentist appointment.
9–10 a.m.	Return books to library. Talk to Melinda in front of library.
10–11 a.m.	Pick up blouse at tailor's. Go to post office for stamps. Buy panty hose.
11–12 p.m.	Have lunch with Julia.
12–1 p.m.	Buy light bulbs. Take car in for wheel alignment. Shop in mall while car is being fixed.
1–2 p.m.	. . . Well, I'm sure you get the idea. This is pretty boring stuff, so I won't ask you to read through the whole day!

43

EMOTIONS

For emotional peace and direction, I can suggest one of two options. If you're a believer, I recommend prayer. Simply say over and over again during the day, "Please, God, help me have a good diet day today." Say it dozens, even hundreds of times, whenever you think of it. Say it even when it seems least likely to help—when you're reaching for something you shouldn't be eating, for example. And don't forget to thank Him if you make it through the day.

44

If you're not a believer, you will find that affirmations can serve the same purpose. Say repeatedly during the day, "I will have a good diet day today." Say it as you drive along, as you watch TV, during whatever you're doing. Say it over and over, whenever the thought crosses your mind.

Again, obsessive behavior, and again, a technique that works.

What do all of these techniques have in common? Essentially, they're activities that make you feel good. Your overeating, your loss of control, have made you feel bad. To counteract this, you must determinedly get involved in things that make you feel better. This defuses the crazy feelings, the panic reactions, the anxiety. To continue wallowing in your misery is likely to make you overeat again.

WHEN ALL ELSE FAILS

There are times, of course, when nothing is of any help. You just can't seem to stop your out-of-control eating. What I recommend at these times (and we all have them) is that you try to control *what* you eat, even if you have no control over how much.

Allow yourself all you want of any fruits and vegetables, even potatoes or dried fruit. This establishes *some* degree of control and usually leads to an improved ability to return to a diet within a few days at most. It may not be a perfect diet, but it's not a *bad* diet either. Overindulging in healthy foods is a major improvement over indulging in unhealthy junk. I'd rather eat a huge box of raisins than one scoop of ice cream, because for people like me, there's no such thing as just one scoop.

45

PRACTICE MAKES PROGRESS

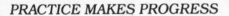

Successful dieting is not an immediate shift; it's a painstaking metamorphosis. You have developed habits you may never be able to conquer, so you must learn to live with them and, to the greatest degree possible, master them. Hopefully, you're making ongoing progress to your goal.

Remember that it's an evolutionary process, not an unblemished pathway to success. Time and again you will have to decide what direction to take, because to be on a diet is not a decision you make only once. You make it over and over again during the course of the diet, and each time there's a battle within yourself to eat. When you falter, you must dust yourself off and pledge your commitment anew—not the commitment to diet perfectly, but the commitment to see it through.

IS THE AMERICAN
BODY IDEAL TOO THIN?

The American ideal of what constitutes attractiveness is getting ever thinner and thinner.

Item: The judges in last year's Miss America Pageant commented that the contestants were thinner than in any previous year. They added that in their opinion, this was a reflection of contemporary society as a whole.

Item: The *Playboy* centerfolds have been getting consistently thinner.

Item: Marilyn Monroe, the sex goddess of her era, was much rounder than today's ideal. As for Mae West, fifty years ago she was the epitome of feminine pulchritude; today she'd be considered decidedly fat.

Of course, the American ideal has nothing to do with American *reality*. If anything, our population is becoming increasingly overweight. This discrepancy between the way we are and the way we're told to be causes unhappiness for millions. We are a nation preoccupied with weight, uncomfortable and unhappy with our bodies. Women in particular are obsessed with their weight, and even the slimmest are always going on a diet.

48

Which brings us to this question: Is the American body ideal too thin? Are we setting standards that are unrealistic, even unhealthy, for ourselves?

Personally, I think not—though I know that's not what you were hoping to hear! I have no problem with the media emphasizing and establishing the thin body as a cultural norm, because this encourages people to strive to be thin—and I believe that to be thin is to be your best.

I am not a subscriber to the "Fat Is Beautiful" school of thought. Fat is *not* beautiful, nor is it healthy. It can destroy both the quality and the duration of your life. It steals your time and your energy, because every second spent thinking about weight, diet and food is a precious moment lost. Almost anything else is more interesting, more edifying and more productive.

I believe that it is to your advantage to get thin enough to put the problem completely behind you for life—so completely that not only is weight not on your body, it is not even on your mind. Imagine being free of this terrible preoccupation!

What, then, is your ideal weight? I do not consider it realistic to assign one inflexible number as a person's "ideal weight." No one stays the same weight day in and day out, not even those who have never had a weight problem. In the normal course of events, we sometimes weigh a pound or two more or a pound or two less, and that is perfectly fine. Indeed, it is inevitable. Perhaps we've been to a party and eaten a bit more than usual. Or we've been so absorbed in a project that we had no time to eat.

49

What makes more sense to me is to assign a *range* of acceptable weights. This is more realistic and less obsessive than having to weigh one particular number. As long as you're anywhere within the acceptable range for your height, you should consider yourself problem-free.

The goal weights I suggest are listed on page 51. Note that the first column reads "Do Not Weigh Less Than," while the second one says "Do Not Weigh More Than." I think it is imperative to provide minimum weights as well as maximum weights. We all know the number we're not supposed to go *above*, but no weight chart has ever told us what we should not go *below*. We need to know the complete parameters of good health and good looks.

In particular, anorexics and bulimics need to know at what point they are, indeed, thin enough. To my mind, the absence of minimum weights has contributed to these two diseases, because dieters have never known when to *stop*. My feeling is that the minimums on my chart are just about as low as one should go, though if you wanted to lose another pound or two, you could do so without endangering your health. But that's *it*—go no lower. The same holds true for the top of the range—a pound or two more won't kill you, but it *can* place you in jeopardy and is therefore best avoided.

50

My recommendation is that you go all the way down to the minimum in order to ascertain where you look and feel your best. In particular, people who have had a serious weight problem should stick to the lower or middle range, since they have a history of excess and should take care to avoid danger. Remember, the weight problem may have been resolved, but the food problem remains, and you'd be wise to keep a few pounds in reserve for the times when you're likely to need them.

Of course, the best reason for getting very thin is that it makes it easier to keep the weight off. People often tell me they don't want to get "too thin." They say, "But I look good when I'm at 140," or "I was happy at 140. I could wear a size 10." They consider these valid reasons for wanting to stop there again, not seeing where their reasoning breaks down.

The point is that they didn't *stay* at 140.

WOMEN			MEN		
	Do Not Weigh Less Than	Do Not Weigh More Than		Do Not Weigh Less Than	Do Not Weigh More Than
4'11"	91	95	5'2"	110	118
5'	94	100	5'3"	115	124
5'1"	97	105	5'4"	120	130
5'2"	100	110	5'5"	125	136
5'3"	104	115	5'6"	130	142
5'4"	108	120	5'7"	135	148
5'5"	112	125	5'8"	140	154
5'6"	117	130	5'9"	145	160
5'7"	122	135	5'10"	150	166
5'8"	127	140	5'11"	155	172
5'9"	132	145	6'	160	178
5'10"	137	150	6'1"	165	184
5'11"	142	155	6'2"	170	190
6'	147	160	6'3"	175	196
			6'4"	180	202
			6'5"	185	208

51

The lower figures on this chart come from Duke University's famous Rice Diet Clinic. The higher figures come from the following standard formula: for women, 100 pounds for the first five feet of height, plus five pounds for every inch over that. For men, it's 106 pounds for the first five feet, and six pounds for each additional inch.

It was just too close to the point where they started to look thick, too close to the treacherous place where they began to put the weight on. What difference does it make how good you looked or what size you wore if you couldn't *stay* there?

You must go past the point where you "look good" to the point where you're *safe.* Even if it means weighing less than you ever considered, less than you really want. Otherwise the whole thing is likely to be an exercise in futility, and you'll soon be fighting the same terrible battle again. You must get so thin that you (almost!) eliminate the danger of putting it back on.

It is true, of course, that you can't weigh this little and eat a whole lot—but we eat too much anyway, virtuously telling ourselves that we "require" 2000 or more calories a day. However, we only "require" such a large number of calories if a lot of those calories are being wasted on non-nutritional foods.

You can eat literally thousands of calories and still not be getting your nutritional needs met if you are selecting the wrong foods. In fact, many overweight people are malnourished because of their poor dietary choices. Lunch at a fast-food restaurant can net you a couple of thousand calories while leaving basic nutritional needs unmet. Yet you can eat as few as 700 calories a day, and if you choose wisely, you'll get all the vitamins, minerals and fiber you need—without taking supplements either.

It is ridiculous and even dangerous to think that we need a substantial number of calories to thrive. We like to eat, so we want to believe this, but quite the contrary is true. In a recent experiment at Cornell University, underfed rats lived 33 percent longer than rats permitted to eat all they wanted. Harvard researchers have found that people who live the longest are those who weigh at least 10 percent less than the average for their height.

53

Those who criticize some healthy diets as being too low in calories are overlooking the fact that more people are in hospitals from eating too much than from eating too little.

If eating sparingly means you're occasionally hungry, where's the problem in that? Opt for good health and safety—opt for eating and weighing less.

CAN YOU TRUST
YOUR BODY'S
MESSAGES?

There is a school of thought that claims our body will let us know what food it needs, and we should trust our body's messages. I subscribe to this theory, but with one important precondition: by all means, trust your body, but only if you've trained it properly first.

A body that has been fed nothing but adulterated foods has no basis of knowledge for sending the appetite the correct signals. An analogy can be made to a computer. Program it with inaccurate information, and it will never be able to turn out correct replies.

Just as our mind needs to be educated in order to fulfill its true potential, our bodies need an appropriate education, too.

Unfortunately, most of us send our bodies to the School of Hard Knocks. From birth on, we batter, burden and torment them with the wrong kinds of food. Mistreated bodies are incapable of telling us what they need, because they themselves have never been fed accurate information.

Like alcohol and drugs, bad food will affect how your mind works; and how can you make the right decisions when you literally can't think straight? As it stands now, your body is working against you. All it knows is the treacherous foods you've been feeding it, so when it tells you it wants to eat, it urges you to reach for the unhealthy foods it is familiar with.

I believe you must rid your body of offending substances before your mind can be unclouded enough to respond rationally. This means retraining your body, and as with all serious undertakings, it will take time. Regard it as a remedial course designed to remove you forever from anxieties about when and how much to eat.

There are two different times when your body sends you messages—before you eat and after you've eaten.

What you feel before you eat is most commonly identified as hunger. It is important that you learn to distinguish between being hungry and just wanting to eat. "I want to eat" is a message *to* your body, while hunger is a valid message *from* it. Remember that wishful thinking is *not* a body message!

This is not to say that you should eat
only when genuinely hungry, which could
make eating a random, inappropriate or
inconvenient affair. We live in a society that
has a clearly structured three-meals-a-day
pattern, and I believe you'd be wise to train
your body to adapt to it. This means pick-
ing three two-hour time spans during the
day, and calling them breakfast, lunch and
dinner. Make sure you eat your allotted
meal sometime during that two-hour period. If you're not particularly hungry, you
should still eat, but choose to eat less. (If
you never eat breakfast, say, or lunch, I
have no problem with that, as long as your
remaining meals are eaten at the same
time daily.)

With the passage of time, you will find
that your body will come to expect to be fed
at certain times—and at those times only.
This will eliminate the craving for between-
meal or nighttime snacks. If you always
have a snack at 9 p.m., even if it's only an
apple, your body is going to demand food
every night at nine, and eventually this
habit is bound to cause you problems.

Where we also have trouble is in *inter-
preting* our body's messages. It's amazing
how often our body demands that we eat
the very thing we happen to want! We have
come to have some kind of magical belief in
the sanctity of our "gut feelings," and for
the life of me, I can't see why. Logic and
common sense are still our best guides.

Let's take a look at the body's *reactions*

to the foods we eat—a very informative type of message.

Losing weight should be regarded as nothing less than a scientific undertaking. It is an experiment that you are performing on your body, your own personal lab. Pay attention to how you feel after you eat the wrong foods, or too much. Notice if you have a reaction to any particular items in your diet. (For example, dairy products often cause the dairy-sensitive to produce mucus, necessitating blowing your nose or clearing your throat after eating them.)

58

Excessive or inappropriate eating is not a pleasant experience for your body, and it will tell you that it feels sluggish, bloated or stiff. Your mental attitude may also be affected, with depression and lethargy very common results.

This is obviously not how you should feel after eating. You should feel "up" after a meal, satisfied and somehow *right*.

By now, my body's messages have become fairly reliable—and it turns out my body wants to eat a healthy, balanced diet. Yours will, too, because that's the nature of the beast. Note that this does not necessarily mean balanced within a specific twenty-four-hour period. For example, sometimes I'm in the mood for potatoes, and will eat them meal after meal for a couple of days. Then suddenly I'll be wanting bananas, or salmon steak, and that's what I'll eat. Over time it evens out.

As long as you limit yourself to plain, unadulterated foods, you will not need to worry about your intake or your weight, and you should feel comfortable responding to your body's messages. However, with each additional category of food that you include, you will be adding another element of distortion. The farther you move from your body's natural diet, the more untrustworthy your body's messages to you will become. You *can* trust your body's messages, but only if your body can trust *you* to treat it well.

59

IS OVERWEIGHT REALLY A PSYCHOLOGICAL PROBLEM?

We've all seen it dozens of times. Someone writes to Ann Landers or Dear Abby requesting help with her weight problem. The answer is always the same: "Get into therapy and find out what's *really* wrong. In order to lose weight, you first have to find out what's causing you to eat."

We're all familiar with these terms: "obsessive-compulsive behavior," "submerged needs," "fears of intimacy and sex." For the overweight, the psychiatrist has become the Court of Last Resort. But exactly how helpful *is* psychological intervention?

It has become fashionable of late to regard excess weight as a psychological problem, but if obesity were psychologically motivated, wouldn't it be responsive to psychological treatment? The fact that psychotherapy has been by and large unsuccessful in this area suggests that other causes must be examined.

I personally believe that the problem is physiological. From birth on, we have been fed nothing but adulterated food. Many suffer from food sensitivities, especially to sugar and salt. Though they may not be aware of it (it's not immediately evident, like a case of hives), these foods stimulate appetite. If you're genetically predisposed this way, it can be painfully easy to put on weight.

62

Excess weight is often evidence of disturbed biological functioning. Despite your determination to diet, your body may actually be working against you—urging you, pressuring you, almost compelling you to eat. Many overweight people don't have "addictive personalities," they have addictive bodies. To say "It's all in your head" is simplistic and unfair.

The problem frequently isn't the person, it's the poison—and in my experience, the culprit is usually salt. As I learned from my experience at Duke University, when you eat salt, you are introducing a chemical— sodium chloride—into your system. If you are sodium-sensitive, it can create an inflammatory reaction—the compulsion to eat.

Some examples: Can you eat just one salted peanut, salted pretzel or salted potato chip? It isn't the nut, grain or potato that makes you crave more, since in their natural state these foods don't have that effect. No, what impels you to keep on eating is unquestionably the stimulating effect of the salt. Confirming evidence can be seen in an Australian study in which two groups of patients were fed exactly the same food, one with salt and one without. The patients in the salt group gained weight, while the others did not.

I believe that cutting out added sodium *in all forms* would permanently eliminate almost all weight problems—and not to worry: you'll still get enough to meet your body's needs. Salt appears naturally in almost everything we eat. Heck, even our tap water is loaded with the stuff!

In stressing the effects of sodium, I am not ruling out the negative effects of other foods. There are many who cannot tolerate sugar or fat, for example, in their diet. But salt in particular triggers a longing for more food, and sets you off.

I urge you to at least try a sodium-free diet to see what this one change can do for you. Certainly it's a preferable option to regarding yourself as nuts! I think you'll discover that the problem is sodium, not the psyche.

Please don't interpret any of the above as a negative appraisal of psychotherapy. I benefited enormously from therapy, and I'm a psychotherapist myself. So I am all in favor of getting psychological help...for psychological problems. Where I have trou-

63

ble is when therapists treat people with *physical* problems as though they were strictly emotional. This is an understandable professional bias, but one that can be harmful to the patient. Most psychiatrists do not even do physical examinations, though qualified to do so, and all too often patients who need nutritional treatment are given drugs.

64

Even behavior modification, once highly touted as a helpful route to weight control, is now largely regarded as a failure in this area. As a technique, it has many successful applications—but not in this particular field. Indeed, many behavioral therapists now refuse to treat obesity, since past experience has shown them that this approach does not help.

By all means, go for therapy, but be aware of its limitations. It *can* change your life in many wonderful ways, but it's unlikely to make you thin.

Regarding overweight as a psychological problem does a great disservice to the dieter. By blaming the victim (who's already miserable), feelings of inadequacy and guilt are produced. It also suggests that the problems are so deep-rooted that in most cases nothing can be done. A shift in perspective can offer relief from self-recrimination—as well as greater likelihood of success.

Though I don't believe that obesity is caused by psychological problems, I do think it can cause such problems. When we feed our bodies properly, these emotional factors fall into place. In other words, we don't need to resolve our emotional problems before we can diet. Instead, if we diet, most emotional problems will disappear. I don't have a fraction of the problems now that I had when I weighed 275!

We readily accept that our minds affect our bodies—no one questions the existence of psychosomatic diseases. Yet we pooh-pooh the notion that our bodies can affect our minds. I dispute this, and urge you to investigate for yourself. Start eating properly and see what a difference this makes in your emotional life. Just a few days of good eating will be enough to tell the tale. What we really need is kitchen therapy, not psychotherapy!

65

OVERWEIGHT AND
DEPRESSION

Much like the chicken and the egg, it is hard to know which comes first—overweight or depression. Certainly they are cyclical and feed (so to speak!) upon each other. You eat because you're depressed; then you get depressed because you ate. The image of the jolly fat person couldn't be farther from the truth.

I'm sure you'll agree that happiness doesn't come from what you have, but from what you are. And if what you are is fat, then it's practically impossible to be happy. Who can look at a picture of Christina Onassis in a bathing suit and envy her her millions?

Improper eating obviously affects our bodies, causing physical problems ranging from tooth decay and hives to diabetes and heart disease. Who can believe that it doesn't affect us psychologically and emotionally as well? This is, of course, compounded by the social stigma of excess weight.

Let's take a look at the four P's that influence depression: Perfectionism, Pain, Psychological readiness and Proper eating.

PERFECTIONISM

Depression can ensue from trying to conform to social norms that are an almost impossible standard of physical perfection. Since we tend to approach our own looks critically, it is usually daunting to compare ourselves with others.

This is an issue with an even greater effect on women, whose incidence of both overweight and depression is significantly higher than men's. Most women are supersensitive to every pound above the norm; many believe they have a weight problem when they don't.

The self-absorption (struggling to be perfect), combined with self-rejection (inevitably failing), leads to anxiety and depression.

Nor, indeed, is it enough for a woman to be thin. There are even more exacting specifics. We're supposed to have large, firm breasts, long, shapely legs, a perfectly oval face—and we'd darn well better be young, too! How can we not end up feeling inferior when we compare ourselves with this ideal?

Take one sobering look at what *real-life* women look like, and forget about trying to be perfect. Aim at being your imperfect best.

PAIN

It's generally acknowledged that when you're depressed, under stress or anxious, you're likely to turn to food for comfort. Of course, that's the very worst time to eat, because it will only make you feel worse than before. Life is more manageable when your eating is under control. Problems are more readily handled, perspective more easily maintained. Food as a source of comfort only leaves you feeling empty and depressed.

69

Among the overweight and depressed, it is a common belief that "things would be better if only I lost weight"—and this is true.

When you're fat, your life, if not worthless, certainly seems worth less to you. A decrease in self-consciousness allows you to focus outside yourself. My main quarrel with overweight is that it is such an inward preoccupation. You tend to look at your navel instead of being involved with life. Your weight becomes your main issue, so that you are both literally and metaphorically absorbed by it.

Many overweight people put their lives on hold, pending the loss of weight. They're waiting to be thin for their "real lives" to begin. If this is true of you, you are wasting your life, and I urge you to stop. What is, shall not be again; enjoy it now, because this is its moment.

PSYCHOLOGICAL READINESS

70

Overweight is a dependent state (you're dependent on food), and dependence leads to depression. Only freedom from addiction will permit you to find happiness. It's much easier to be happy when your eating is under control, and so damn hard to be happy when it isn't. Everything looks better when *you* do—so what are you waiting for?

Ah, I know! You're waiting to be psychologically ready! This is one of my favorites. Why, I'd like to know, *in this one area only,* is it all right to wait until you're psychologically ready before you'll do what must be done? For example, you need to support yourself, so you go to work; you don't wait till you're psychologically ready to get a job. And if exams are around the corner, you study *now;* you don't wait till you're psychologically ready to hit the books. Nor, I'll bet, do you ask the IRS to wait till you're psychologically ready to pay your taxes. You darn well get that check in by April 15. With weight, however, there is no compelling external force to make us do what we must do.

Contemporary society reveres "feelings," but to my mind, doing is much more important. Doing provides results, while heeding our "feelings" can be fruitless self-indulgence and a downright waste of time.

PROPER EATING

In truth, the change in your life will come not so much from being thin, but from choosing to eat properly on a consistent basis. Yes, part of your depression is a result of being overweight, but a much larger proportion is being caused by the foods you eat. Unnatural, processed, salty and sugary foods contribute to your depression. Eat plain, natural foods and you will see a radical difference in your mood. Moreover, you will see these results immediately, virtually within a few days.

71

It is not just the loss of weight, it is healthy food itself that will bring you serenity. Getting thin may be your long-term goal, but there will be payoffs from Day One.

THE FORTUNE FACTOR

*The Part Luck Plays
in Weight Loss*

When I first lost weight, I asked Dr. Kempner if he thought I would ever gain it back. "No problem," he said. "You are too curious about life to gain your weight back." He then added, "One just has to hope that you don't have too much bad luck in life."

This is a very interesting perspective. Weight loss is usually seen as completely within the individual's control—which is one of the reasons there is so much guilt and blame attached to excess weight.

The fact is, however, that not everything is within our control. We try to diet in the context of the ongoing events in our lives, and sometimes these events—our "luck," if you will—can render a diet virtually impossible. Let me give you some examples:

One day I met a former Rice Diet patient at the Rice House. Eight years earlier, she had dieted down to 128 pounds and had kept the weight off all that time. Then the last year she regained it all. Appalled (are you *never* safe?), I asked what had caused her to gain the weight back after all those years. She told me that in the course of one year, her husband left her, her mother died, she had a breast removed due to cancer (which later turned out not to be malignant!) and her son committed suicide. Obviously, counting calories was the last thing on her mind.

74

Another woman told me that she had a hard time sticking with a diet because her husband liked to eat out a lot. I self-righteously told her that her needs were as great as his and she should just refuse to accompany him. Well, it turns out that her husband is blind, and unless she drives him to a restaurant, he cannot go. This changes things entirely, of course. She doesn't feel right refusing him one of his few remaining pleasures just because she can't control her appetite.

It is important to look at your willingness and ability to diet in the context of your total life. Dieting is not done in a vacuum, and it can be an impossible undertaking if your life is crashing down around your ears. There are times that are better or worse for us to start, and there are times when it's a virtual impossibility.

When considering starting a diet, first evaluate how much power you have at that particular moment. You might find yourself saying, "Wow. All these things are happening now." It is next to impossible to undertake two major projects at the same time, and dieting is a hard enough endeavor when there's no other problem in sight.

It is understandable that when your world falls apart, food appears to offer some solace, if not a solution. If this describes your situation, don't be critical and punitive with yourself. Recognize that the time for dieting may not be now.

Of course, we both know that eating doesn't solve your problems; it makes them worse. Indeed, eating properly helps us take our problems in stride. But that is logic, and it can be hard to live in a rational way when hit with emotional devastation. There are times when misfortune has us in its grip.

This is not the time to flagellate yourself because you can't stick with a diet. Luck plays a part in virtually all aspects of our lives. We must be careful not to exempt weight loss from its powerful effects.

THE CHEATER'S
REPORT CARD

Being all-or-nothing by nature, dieters are usually either rigidly ON a diet or else chaotically OFF. We know no shades of gray. One bite beyond what a diet permits often serves as the start of a binge. ("What the heck, I've already broken the diet anyway.") If we're not on the perfect diet, then we're running amok.

This usually makes us even fatter, leading to the increasingly popular theory that "diets don't work." Of course they do, if *you* will work at them. And "working at them" doesn't mean being the Perfect Dieter, as desirable as that may be.

I believe that it is imperative that we redefine success and failure. We need to find a middle ground between perfection and total loss of control. I would therefore like to suggest various fallback positions. In essence, cheating must be placed in a structured framework that permits the dieter to cheat, yet still adhere to the diet to some degree.

The premise is taken from the old grade-school report cards, which used to evaluate us as follows:

E	Excellent
VG	Very Good
G	Good
F	Fair
U	Unsatisfactory

78

How is this applied to diet?

Well, an E day is obviously one in which our diets are absolutely flawless.

A VG day is one in which a dieter cheats with small extra quantities of the foods she or he is allowed on the diet anyway (e.g., extra fruit, another baked potato or piece of chicken).

A day rates a G when you've eaten only permissible foods, but in excessive quantities.

An F day is one in which you eat small quantities of nonpermissible foods (an ice-cream cone, a chocolate bar, etc.).

A day is Unsatisfactory only when you've completely gone off the deep end.

Naturally, you should aim for as high a "grade" as possible, but a good deal of latitude is allowed before a day should be regarded as a failure.

To permit cheating options within a certain reasonable range relieves you of the unrealistic pressure to be perfect, and removes the guilt that accompanies even the slightest transgression. Knowing that all is not necessarily lost just because you had something extra can help avert an all-out binge. It puts the whole issue in a more reasonable context.

There are other advantages as well. Over a period of time, you will see certain patterns emerge, and it can be of value to know how many days of the month fall into each of these categories. How many days do you binge, and on how many days are you perfect? Are you fairly consistent, or are there some good months and some total write-offs? And what does that mean in terms of your weight?

79

When I was dieting, I found this perspective helpful because each time I binged I tended to panic. Was this the end of my ability to diet? Was I on my way back up to 275? If I could look back and see that I routinely binged four or five times a month, yet continued to lose, I could feel reassured that this new binge was probably in the same category—a relatively isolated incident and not the thin (so to speak!) edge of the wedge. I had a recorded history that demonstrated that a binge was nothing more than an occasional lapse, not a sign of doom. It had happened before; it would, alas, happen again.

On the following page is a blank sample

of a Report Card for your use. I strongly recommend it as a means of putting the issue into perspective. A successful dieter is not perfect—she or he operates on a continuum. Such gradations of acceptable dieting can help you stick with it over the long haul.

80

MONTH	E	VG	G	F	U
	——days	——days	——days	——days	——days
	——days	——days	——days	——days	——days
	——days	——days	——days	——days	——days
	——days	——days	——days	——days	——days
	——days	——days	——days	——days	——days
	——days	——days	——days	——days	——days
	——days	——days	——days	——days	——days

CAN YOU EXPECT OTHERS TO LOVE YOU "JUST THE WAY YOU ARE"?

I know just how the reasoning goes: "If someone really cares about me, they shouldn't care about my appearance, but should accept me just as I am, for the person I am."

But exactly how valid is this? Unfortunately, most often it's a romantic fantasy. The truth is that most normal-weight people react to the overweight with the instinctive withdrawal usually reserved for reptiles. Excess weight distracts others from seeing us positively, especially at an initial meeting. Many never get past their unfavorable first impression. Indeed, even fat people themselves are prejudiced against the overweight.

As a nation, we pay lip service to the idea that true beauty lies within, but in reality we virtually worship an attractive exterior. Appearance makes a real difference in dozens of daily encounters, with the attractive getting preferential treatment in school, in relationships and on the job. This fact may be seen as reprehensible, but it cannot be denied.

Appearance even makes a difference in how others respond to one's opinions and ideas. For example, after the first Nixon-Kennedy debate, the majority of those who heard it on the radio thought that Nixon had won the debate, while those who *saw* it on TV were convinced that Kennedy was the clear winner. More proof, if any was needed, that we live in a very visual age.

The importance of appearance can lead to pain and humiliation for the overweight. I still remember the time I went to a new hairdresser and waited for over an hour before the embarrassed receptionist told me that "Monsieur Pierre refuses to do you."

This attitude goes beyond real hurts and imagined slights to actual discrimination, especially on the job. Did you know that, except in the State of Michigan, it is actually legal to discriminate on the basis of size?

The overweight are also the butt of hurtful jokes. Comics can stand on a national stage and make remarks that wound and offend a significant number of people in their audience. Yet no one complains—indeed, the overweight themselves often laugh the loudest. They don't believe they have the right to complain; they feel too guilty, responsible and defenseless.

Excessive weight is considered unappetizing and unseemly—an opinion often shared even by our nearest and dearest.

Notice how often weight gained after marriage causes arguments and acrimony. The spouse often feels that he's a victim of the old "bait and switch." It is possible that your kids will feel embarrassed, too, if you're substantially overweight.

83

Of course, this issue will affect your relationships for more reasons than the simply visual. When your eating is out of control, especially when the excess includes (as it usually does) unhealthy foods, your emotional state will be affected, and with it, your ability to relate. The agitation, depression and anxiety caused by poor eating will inevitably affect other aspects of your life.

Obviously, you have diminished resources to give others when you're self-preoccupied and not feeling your best. Overeating frequently leads to self-hatred —and if we're incapable of loving ourselves, how can we expect others to love us?

Which brings us to our original question: *Can* you expect others to love you "just the way you are"? Quite frankly, I think not.

An agreeable appearance is part of what we contribute to our relationships, and it is unfair to regard others as insensitive or superficial just because they include an attractive exterior among their needs. Whether it's furniture, clothing or mates, aesthetic appeal invariably counts.

Somehow, even "inner beauty" seems more visible when you're thin. Your character, intelligence and personality may be appreciated, but most likely they'll be negated or overlooked if you're overweight. What's the good of having everything going for you if you're unable to make it work for you?

To claim that things "shouldn't" be this way is to demand unconditional love. This is something that all of us long for, of course, but, alas, it's neither reasonable nor realistic. It may be a bitter pill to swallow, but most people will *not* love you just as you are.

YOUR DIET/YOUR FAMILY: WHOSE RIGHTS SHOULD PREVAIL?

It is difficult enough to stay on a diet at the best of times—and those who have to shop for and prepare food for others have an especially difficult row to hoe. Someone living alone may have to deal with temptations, but those living in a family context have additional difficulties to face.

To have unpermitted food within arm's reach is asking too much of the dieter, and I therefore believe that a special "diet time" should be put aside. During this period, no nondiet foods should be permitted in the house. There should be nothing but fruits, vegetables, grains (and grain products), chicken, fish and eggs on the premises.

I know, I can hear you from here. What about my husband's favorite, or the treats for my kids? Surely it isn't fair to ask them to give up those things.

No? And why not? It's even less fair to ask you to fight off the urge, especially when it's critically important for you to lose weight.

I believe that it is unfair to expose loved ones trying to diet to foods that will cause them to fall off their chosen path. Surely everything possible should be done to make your task easier, not harder. Anyone can forgo pizza, ice cream or pretzels for the period of time it takes you to reach your weight-loss goals.

Nor, indeed, do they have to do without their favorite snacks—you are just asking them not to eat them in the house, where you are exposed to the sights and smells. What's unfair about that? Yours is a question of health, theirs a matter of whim. Those junk foods they want aren't doing *them* any good either!

It can be argued that I am being unrealistic. Perhaps so. The fact is, this is not my own situation. I live alone, and perhaps I greatly underestimate the problems involved in turning a whole household over into a diet house.

Well, I may not know what dieting in a family situation is like, but I *do* know the power of food, and I don't see how anyone with even a relatively serious weight problem (say, thirty pounds or more) can man-

age to stay on a diet while having to
consistently see, shop for, prepare, smell,
handle and live with food. It is hard
enough without the ever-present temptation. When you experience that moment of
craving, that sudden desire, compulsion,
yearning for food—if all you have to do is
reach out and a second later it is in your
mouth—well, I wish you the best of luck,
but I think your efforts will be severely
jeopardized.

Bad food is our enemy, and your loved
ones must somehow be made to understand that. You must do whatever you can
to make the situation as problem-free as
possible, and your loved ones should be
willing to help. It would be nice if they were
downright *happy* to help, and in loving
families this will be the case.

You must ask your family to be your support system—which does not mean being
your baby-sitter or your warden. They
should not be asked to *make* you stay on a
diet, only to help. Get them involved in
buying and preparing food; have someone
else clear up after meals. In particular, ask
them not to talk about food, because you
know how discussions about food can be
lethal.

The overweight tend to think very little
of themselves, and it can be hard for them
to make such demands. They feel guilty if
they think of putting themselves first. But
this is not just for you. Your eating problems cannot help but affect your family.

Inappropriate eating invariably affects your mood and your behavior. It leads to anxiety, depression, withdrawal or aggressiveness. You can be so absorbed by your own misery that you're desensitized to others' needs. Unhealthy eating damages your ability to relate to the outside world. You're focused inward, you're focused on pain—and when you're unhappy, you have much less to give. Physically, too, you're unable to do as much. Going on a diet is a favor you do for *everyone*.

SABOTEURS AND
SUPPORTERS

Excess pounds are unquestionably a personal tragedy for the overweight, but others in your life can be affected as well. Some may have genuine concerns about your health and happiness; others may be threatened by a change in the status quo. The former will want to help you; the latter may try to sabotage. Either way, the dieter can't help but be affected by the input of others.

This chapter is intended to be read by those with weight problems and by those who are close to someone with a weight problem. I have broken it down into two sections—those who hinder and those who help.

THOSE WHO HINDER

It is not always true that others want you to lose weight. Sabotage can come from the most unexpected sources. A saboteur can be your best friend, your mother or your husband—someone who ostensibly cares about you the most. And indeed they may care, but they can't help but be subject to mixed motives as well. Relationships are complex, and we all have our areas of craziness.

Sabotage is not necessarily all ill will; indeed, it is often unconscious behavior. The saboteur doesn't always know what he or she is doing, and would deny wanting anything for you but the best. Nonetheless, nutsiness can prevail. A close relative of mine, someone who would be truly distraught if I were to gain weight, has been known to a) ask me to buy her a bag of chocolate chip cookies, knowing that they're one of my few remaining weaknesses; b) hide them from me (which I certainly don't ask her to do); then c) wonder out loud if I can find them. (I just say, "I'm not even going to look," and let it drop.) Habits die hard, and many families have crazy behavior patterns around food.

Another woman told me her husband nags her incessantly about losing weight, then routinely brings home her favorite pastries, telling her curtly to "show a little willpower." He obviously *doesn't* mean so well, and her weight is only one of the sore points in this marriage.

Another common saboteur is the "binge-ing buddy," the person you often share eating experiences with. These friends may initially be supportive, but as you succeed in losing weight, they can turn against you. Saboteurs will talk lovingly about food; they will offer you something to eat ("A little isn't going to hurt"); they will accuse you of being a fanatic or they will tell you you're starting to look gaunt.

To my mind, anyone who knows that you are struggling with a food problem and nonetheless offers you food is offering you poison. These people aren't considering your feelings or your needs, and you should feel no sense of obligation toward them.

Of course, it is necessary to distinguish between the merely hospitable and the saboteur. It requires one kind of approach not to "hurt your hostess's feelings," and still another to deal with a "friend" who repeatedly brings over cookies. I look at it this way: if someone offers me food once, I regard it as politeness. Twice, and I become a little chilly. Three times, and I scratch him off my list.

Naturally, you must make it clear right from the start that you're trying to lose weight and don't want to be offered food. The responsibility for getting your needs met must be yours. You must speak up, make demands and stick to your guns, come what may. This is an issue of assertiveness, the kind of openness required to make others aware of your needs.

Weight loss is a process requiring various forms of self-development and growth. Dealing with the pressures and mixed motives of others can definitely be a challenge. The physical changes one makes by losing weight are almost invariably matched by profound changes on the personal level. Handling sabotage may be an important problem to be resolved.

92

THOSE WHO HELP

This section is intended for the person who genuinely wants to help an overweight loved one but doesn't know how.

Excess weight is a very sensitive and personal issue, and frequently, not even those closest to you dare broach the subject. Often the overweight person gives off a sense of the topic being taboo. This can make one's friends nervous, afraid of saying or doing the wrong thing.

The overweight person feels that her normal-weight friends don't really understand—and this is, in fact, true. Nonetheless, there are some guidelines that may help.

DON'T analyze your friend's behavior or background in an effort to find out why she eats. If she wanted therapy, she would consult a professional.

DON'T cut out every article you see on

the topic of weight and hand it to your friend. If you come across something you think she really should be made aware of, say, "I occasionally see articles about weight in the magazines I read. Do you want me to cut them out for you?" Make this offer just once, then guide yourself accordingly.

DON'T offer advice about what to eat or how to lose weight. It amazes me that so many normal-weights think the overweight don't *know* which foods are fattening, and will solemnly advise you to cut out ice cream, French fries and cookies. Believe me, most overweight people know the calorie content of every bite they eat. They know what they should eat and what is fattening. The problem is not one of ignorance of the facts.

DON'T make comments like, "You don't really need that," or "Remember your diet." Statements like these provoke resentment, anger and the feeling that "I'll do as I damn well please."

DON'T try to induce guilt or shame. Your friend feels bad enough without your help, I assure you.

DON'T get into an open confrontation about weight. This is far likelier to lead to a binge than to good results. No amount of yelling or complaining is going to work. Bottom line, the issue is none of your business.

DON'T try scare tactics, like showing your friend clippings about how excess weight can cause disease. She knows, and is plenty worried.

DON'T suggest that your friend join a weight-loss group. Yes, they can help, but she already knows about them, and your suggestion will only be seen as an intrusion.

94

If you invite your friend over, DON'T keep food around in visible areas. DON'T offer her anything but coffee or tea. DON'T ever tell her that "just a little won't hurt." One little taste can trigger a craving, tap into an addiction and set off a binge. Realize that food is something your friend just can't handle.

DON'T eat tempting foods in front of a friend trying to diet.

DON'T talk about food—the mere mention of it can weaken resolve. Would you talk lyrically about liquor in front of a recovering alcoholic? If your friend starts to talk about food, change the subject without being obvious.

DON'T suggest meeting at a restaurant or coffee shop. Instead, when you get together, suggest healthy, enjoyable activities in which food is not part of the pleasure.

DON'T reward a friend with food for doing so well on her diet. Such "treats" are highly inappropriate and even suspect.

Quite a long list of "don'ts." Is there anything you *can* do? Only one thing, really, and that's to let your friend know that you're there.

Love and understanding from family and

friends are particularly important when you're dieting and feeling deprived. Let your loved one know that you're available for support or just for helping pass the time, especially during those difficult first few days. Be prepared to accept that they may not be all that much fun to be around at this time—as with quitting smoking, withdrawal from food can cause a foul mood.

Remain supportive of your loved one as a person. Let them know that you love them and will continue to love them, no matter what they weigh. You stand to accomplish more by strengthening their ego than by judging them and finding them wanting.

95

The best way to approach the subject is to say to your friend, "I know I cannot really understand this problem, but if there is any way I can be of help, please let me know." At least you will have opened the door to discussion. Make your offer forthrightly, make it sincerely—and make it *once*. Despite the best of intentions, this is all you can do.

SEXUAL IMPLICATIONS

At 275 pounds, I had a lot of good reasons for wanting to lose weight, but most compelling among them was the desire to be more attractive to men. Let's face it, you don't often see an overweight woman on the arm of a hunk. Like it or not, looks matter a lot to most men.

Just check the Personals ads that they write. No matter what other qualities they are seeking, no matter how diverse their interests, one thing they all agree on—they want someone slim.

Men are often very intolerant of overweight women; they seem repelled and even find it hard to show any compassion. Terms like "pig" and "slob" express how they feel.

Women, though less stringent, also prefer not to date overweight men. They like their men strong and muscular, not soft and round. They may yearn for a man to take care of them, but they perceive fat men as being able to do this only in a motherly, nonsexual way. Nice to cuddle up to, maybe, but not the stuff of sexual dreams.

Oh, sure, there are "chubby-chasers," men and women who prefer the overweight and seek them out. But they are few and far between, and anyway, isn't there something a little off-putting about being wanted specifically *because* you're overweight?

On the whole, to be overweight is to be a pariah with the opposite sex, although practically everyone numbers at least one overweight person among their same-sex friends. When it comes to love and sex, however, most want someone of average size. As a result, the overweight usually have a vastly diminished social life—and are often too insecure and defensive to try for more. Those who are single find it harder to get dates and sexual partners; the married ones find that even their spouses are often turned off.

The effects of excess weight on sex go beyond the issue of appeal: there can be an actual changing of physical characteristics among the overweight. Overweight women become hairier, especially on the face. This gives them a much more masculine appearance. And everyone is familiar with the overweight man who develops breasts. The more excess weight is carried, the more these lines will blur.

Worse still is the possible development of high blood pressure or diabetes, since medications for these diseases frequently cause impotence in men and decreased libido in women.

And these are just the physical effects of excess weight. The emotional consequences are even more debilitating. It's hard enough to be overweight when dressed in your most flattering attire; to be overweight and *naked* can be unbearably mortifying. This is particularly true when undressing before someone new for the very first time.

99

Insecurity about your appearance is an enormously inhibiting factor. You may be as sensual as all get-out, but if you're concerned about your body, you'll find it hard to let yourself go.

For example, few overweight people feel comfortable making love with the lights on; even in the dark, many refuse to completely undress. Once the act is over, they feel even more exposed and vulnerable. ("Now he's no longer caught up in making love to me. He's going to notice my thighs!")

Certain positions cause heightened self-consciousness; some may even be totally out of the question. Sex becomes fraught with so much anxiety that it can be tough to have a good time.

Losing weight offers you freedom from these sexual limitations. You'll be able to relax and be loving, instead of inwardly agonizing about how you look.

MUST YOU EXERCISE
IN ORDER TO
LOSE WEIGHT?

101

First off, let me say that I think exercise is terrific for you. There is no question—it can lower your blood pressure, tone up your muscles and even alleviate depression. It's a wonderful tool, and I fully endorse it. I never do it, however, because I just darn well don't like to.

Please don't misunderstand me. I am not suggesting that you do not exercise. On the contrary, I think you should. I think *I* should, too, but I have simply never enjoyed it. Short of falling in love with a jock, I'm most unlikely to change my mind.

I bring this up because the prevailing dogma is that unless you exercise, you stand no chance of losing weight. This is simply not true, and I think it is time that someone said so. I lost 140 pounds in nine months and have remained a size 4 for five years without ever doing any exercise. That's right—NONE.

Oh, my first few weeks in Durham, I followed my doctor's recommendations and did a little swimming, but at the earliest opportunity I found an excuse not to continue, and I have done nothing ever since. The fact is, if you're following a good diet, you can do nothing more strenuous than turn the pages of a novel and you will still easily lose weight.

102

I think we do a disservice to the prospective dieter by telling him that not only must he cut down on his beloved food, he must embark on a detested exercise program as well. These double demands, for someone unused to either, can be counterproductive and daunting. To undertake not one but *two* things that you don't much want to do can deter you from even starting. ("What? Not only live on carrot sticks but also run, swim and jog three hours a day??? To heck with that!")

Despite my own abhorrence of physical movement, there are two forms of exercise you may actually enjoy. Even *I* like to do them every once in a while!

The first is walking, which can hardly be called "exercise," since it is the body's natural movement. Walking can be done anywhere, anytime, and it costs you absolutely nothing. It requires no special equipment (except a good pair of shoes, which is a must), and it is easy on the joints. It is good for the entire body and is safe for almost everyone, regardless of age or fitness level.

From my point of view, the best thing about walking is that every time you go out, you expose yourself to involvement with life. You meet people and pets, see both natural and man-made beauties. You hear interesting sounds and conversations and smell all kinds of wonderful smells. If you do decide to start walking, begin slowly; then if you want to, increase distance and time. Never "go for the burn"—in fact, pain during exercise should be regarded as a warning. A stress test is recommended if you're over thirty-five and/or have led a sedentary life.

103

Stretching is another good choice for the relatively inactive. It can help your muscle tone, elasticity, mass and endurance. It feels wonderful, too. I have to admit I actually enjoy it.

I do what I call the "Red Light Stretch." I turn off all the lights, except for one lamp with a red light bulb in it. I turn the radio on to one of those "light" music stations, then stand naked in front of a full-length mirror. I start to move free-form to the music, stretching my arms, legs, whatever, in any direction that feels good. I don't do anything specific; I let my body do what it wants. There are no right or wrong movements, so no two sessions are ever the same. I move slowly, to the limit of the stretch, never forcing myself past the point where I feel comfortable, and I'll keep this up for fifteen or twenty minutes. I set no standards, have no set routines and put no pressure on myself to perform.

I realize that this "red light" description makes the whole procedure sound rather erotic—and indeed it is. Stretching feels so sensuous and so wonderful that I find it difficult to regard it as exercise. But it relaxes and loosens your body, and reverses the atrophying process as well. Some research has even shown that stretching the back—arching it and straightening it—can stop or reverse the loss of calcium from the vertebrae. Stretching also elevates your mood and enhances your overall health.

104

So there *are* ways to keep your body fit without undertaking an extraordinarily ambitious program. We dieters tend to be an all-or-nothing breed, and we usually try to do too much too soon. As with our New Year's resolutions, we decide we're not only going on a diet, at the same time we're going to start exercising, stop smoking, cut down on drinking and stop biting our nails. Needless to say, one small, inevitable slip in any area, and the whole project goes down the tubes.

Being grandiose about exercise is likely to lead to dropping it altogether. You're better off doing moderate exercise over the long haul—which is what the human body was designed for, anyway.

If you decide to exercise (and despite my

own lethargy, I hope you do), set yourself modest goals and work up from there. If you choose not to exercise, don't feel doomed to remain overweight. As beneficial as exercise may be for you, it is NOT a requirement for you to lose weight.

105

OVERCOMING TEMPTATION

You want to lose. But you also want to eat. Okay, what now?

The reasons we give ourselves for eating are varied. Perhaps we're bored. Or under stress. Hey, we may even be hungry (though usually not). Different situations can push our buttons at different times. Let's look at some of the reasons people give for inappropriate eating.

"I'M BORED."

To quote Liz Taylor, "If your mind isn't occupied, then your mouth usually is." Ours is a culture that seeks constant distraction of various kinds, and eating is one of our most popular forms of entertainment. Food is so ubiquitous, so accessible, so immediately satisfying—and, unfortunately, so destructive to you.

"I'VE GOT PROBLEMS."

Eating is often used as a release from tension. However, there is no problem that eating ever made better; it only made it worse. Trying to solve your problems by eating is like trying to put out a fire by pouring on gasoline.

108

"I'M HUNGRY."

Sure you are, and I'm the Queen of Siam. The fact is that few people with weight problems are ever genuinely hungry. They *want to eat*—but that's an entirely different issue. In this country, hunger is happily very rare. Our problems stem from eating too much, not too little. We don't feel we've had enough until, in fact, we've had too much.

We're mistaken in thinking we shouldn't stop eating until we're full. And for many, even "full" isn't enough. I once appeared on the *Phil Donahue* show with the doctor who developed the gastric bubble. This is a balloon device that is inserted (at great cost) down your throat and into your stomach. Once in place, it is blown up and is supposed to make you feel full. I'm sure it does—but what does feeling full have to do with anything? Most people with food problems feel full long before they stop eating. Our bodies have had enough well before our appetites are ready to quit.

What we want is to *eat,* and that should not be confused with hunger. It is important for us to learn to differentiate between the two.

"IT TASTES SO GOOD. I LOVE FOOD AND I LOVE TO EAT."

This one is often accompanied by the feeling that if you don't eat this food *now,* you may never have the chance to eat it again. Perhaps you're at a wedding or a party, or you're in a restaurant or out of town. This is a once-in-a-lifetime opportunity! If you don't taste it now, the opportunity will pass you by.

109

Well, so be it, friend. Being thin tastes even better. Food is always going to taste good, and there will always be something new and different to try. To eat something because it tastes good is to sell your birthright (genuine fulfillment and happiness) for, quite literally, a mess of pottage.

Abstinence pays off more than indulgence does, if what you indulge in causes you pain. Contrary to what you're hoping for, indulgence leads to turmoil more frequently than to pleasure. Especially since most people with a weight problem eat well past the point of enjoyment; they eat to the point of discomfort and anxiety-provoking excess.

So much for the reasons we give ourselves. We tell ourselves we'll start a diet again (fresher! stronger!) tomorrow—or Monday, or after the holidays, or when we get back from our trip.

Logic can only tell you it will not be any easier the next time. Regardless of what diet you're following, the desire to eat is bound to surface again. If you are ever to succeed at losing, at some point you'll have to tell yourself No.

110

To jettison the diet completely is to leave the problem unresolved. If you're like most of us, you will never reach the point of saying to yourself, "To heck with it. I'll just stay fat." Neither our society nor your mind-set will permit you to accept that as an option. This means you'll be primed and ready for the next miracle diet that comes along—the newest and easiest diet, the one that will finally work for you. Only no diet will ever work *for* you. It is *you* who must do all the work.

There's no such thing as an easy diet, because the person who has to diet is the very person who likes to eat. It makes no difference at all *why* you're eating. You'll have one reason today, another tomorrow. It's what you *do* about it that counts. Accordingly, here are some suggestions:

MAJOR ADVICE #1

There is one main technique I use to overcome temptation, and I'll tell you the story about how I learned it.

One morning I went into the Rice House, weighed myself and registered a well-deserved gain. I flopped down on Dr. Gaffron's cot to have my blood pressure taken and started to complain. "I can't help it," I moaned. "Sometimes I almost *have* to eat. I can't seem to stop myself. What should I do?"

Dr. Gaffron leaned over and said softly, "I have the answer. Whenever you want to eat..." Then she paused.

I leaned forward excitedly. This was it! At last I was going to get The Answer. Dr. Gaffron had been working with the overweight for more than forty years. If anyone knew, it was she!

"Whenever you want to eat," she repeated, "do something else instead."

Well, I'm sure you're feeling as disappointed as I felt then. What kind of advice was that? Silly, simplistic advice! But she was right. The best way to keep from eating is to do something else instead. And it doesn't much matter what.

When you feel that you just *have* to eat, recognize that you really don't. You *can* do something else, and you must at least *try* to divert your attention.

Know that the desire to eat, although torturous, is momentary. It comes out of nowhere and it can disappear just as fast. *If* you're willing to let it.

I suggest you draw up a list of things you like to do and consult it when you feel the yearning to break your diet. Include activities that take only a minute or two and others that take several hours. Before you let yourself eat, force yourself to do just one thing on that list.

MAJOR ADVICE #2

112

Even better than having to work at overcoming temptation is choosing to avoid it altogether. We feed our desire to eat by the emphasis we place on food. The path to freedom is through detaching yourself from that passion.

What I am suggesting is that you work at distancing yourself from your love of food. To do this is not hard, but it does take willingness, effort and time.

What you must do is stop indulging all your senses in your inappropriate love of food. Stop reading restaurant reviews, recipe books, food ads and articles about cooking. Don't look at the menu when you eat out—just order what you're allowed. When at a party, don't go over to see what your hostess is serving, even if you swear you're "not going to touch a thing."

Most important of all, DON'T TALK ABOUT FOOD. If others do, change the subject. I always have a hard time convincing people that this matters. They can't see how they can gain weight just by talking about food. Let me assure you, nothing is easier. Talking about food brings it to mind, arouses a craving where none was before. It is like seeing food ads on TV—

you weren't even thinking about it...now you absolutely have to have it. Don't let the process start.

(I have a feeling I'm hearing you say, "Oh, but..." to this one. I would remind you that "but" spelled backward is "tub." Keep talking about food, and I guarantee you that you'll remain tubby!)

To allow yourself to even *think* about food is to buy back into that pain. You may ask, "How can I stop myself from thinking about something?" and to some extent you're right. Thoughts *do* come unbidden into our minds. But we have the power to stop them there. As soon as you're aware that your mind is on food, you can and you must stop it from taking over. It's those second and successive thoughts that compel you to eat. They *can* be avoided if you cooperate with yourself at that point.

113

The trick is to immediately turn your mind to something else. It doesn't have to be anything significant. Look at a nearby tree, the sky, a passerby's shoes. Listen to the cars driving by or turn the radio on. This moment is critical. Do not allow your mind to dwell on food, not even for a second, no matter how tantalizing and seductive it may be. Don't let the thought of food get a foothold in your mind; put your attention quickly on virtually anything else.

Bear in mind that at this moment you are not going to feel like cooperating. Much as you want to lose weight, at that moment what you want to do is eat. But difficult as it may be to force your attention elsewhere, it is much easier than keeping away from food once you have started to crave it. It's also a lot easier than going through life fat.

The first step to acquiring personal power is to distance yourself from whatever it is that weakens you. The second step is to take advantage of whatever will bring you strength.

114

MINI ADVICE

On Eating as a Solution for Boredom

1. I find it helpful to keep several prerecorded VCR tapes on hand so that I always have something distracting to watch. Particularly good are reruns of *The Mary Tyler Moore Show, Rhoda, All in the Family* and *Taxi*. There's nothing like a laugh to get your mind off food. Keep several hours' worth stockpiled for whenever you're at loose ends.

2. Light reading can be a help. Magazines such as *Cosmopolitan* and *People*, weeklies like the *Star* and the *National Enquirer*, all provide diverting and nondemanding reading. Avoid the women's magazines that feature articles on cooking and food.

3. Undertake to do one new thing a day, from trying a new imported fruit to driving down an unfamiliar street to watching a TV show you've never seen. Anything at all that could possibly inter-

est you. Develop your curiosity and appetite for life instead of food.

4. I wonder if any studies have been done linking people with weight problems to those who identify themselves as "night people." This would make sense, because most people who overeat for entertainment tend to do so at night. If this describes you, it is a lifestyle that's to your disadvantage.

   You *can* reset your body clock, and if you eat at night, I suggest you do. Simply start getting up earlier in the morning, which will make you tired earlier at night. Making this change can take from several weeks to a couple of months, but it's very much worth doing if nighttime eating is a problem for you.

5. Another thing night eaters can try is scheduling their dinners later. If you customarily eat at six, then find yourself back at the fridge by nine, try eating your dinner at seven or eight o'clock instead. If this makes it too long between lunch and dinner, have a glass of juice or a piece of fruit or a baked potato in between.

On Eating as a Solution for Problems

You know yourself this never works. Certainly your problems are real, but they will still be there tomorrow. If not one problem, then surely another, because that's the way it is in life. If you consider problems as a valid reason for eating, then that is how you'll spend your life. I'd like to suggest some alternatives:

116

1. Try relaxation techniques. Sit in a comfortable chair or lie down, close your eyes and totally relax your body. Start with your toes, saying to yourself, "Be still, toes." Then move slowly up your entire body. ("Be still, feet. Be still, ankles.") When you get to your face, do each feature separately, including your teeth and tongue. Next command each internal organ to be still. ("Be still, heart. Be still, intestines. Be still, lungs.") Focus your attention on each body part you mention. The most important one, and the one to be kept till last, is "Be still, brain"—because that's where the turmoil originates.

   Once you are relaxed, keep lying still until the urge to eat has passed. I won't say this always works, but more often than not it does.

2. Sometimes, of course, you're in a place where a complete relaxation technique is impossible. At those times, you can get a quick release of tension by completely relaxing all the muscles in your face. This can be done anywhere, anytime.

3. Keep your environment as tranquil as possible. Don't listen to loud and fast music. Don't watch violence on TV. Keep your home and office neat, because disorganization disturbs one's peace of

mind. When at home, don't feel you have to answer the phone. Keep away from negative people and those who live harmful or sordid lives. Do what you must to surround yourself with serenity and beauty.

On Eating Because You're Hungry

Often when we think we're hungry, we're mistaking a whim for a need. And how often "need" turns to greed!

Of course, there are times when it's reasonable and appropriate to be hungry, such as for dinner or lunch. It is important to use a legitimate mealtime as an occasion to move yourself from the desire for food to a feeling of "I've had enough." This is done by selecting foods that satisfy the appetite, not foods that stimulate it.

117

A good, filling diet will be one made up chiefly of fruits, grains and vegetables. These bulky complex carbohydrates quickly make you feel full. Some suggestions:

1. A baked potato and one or two pieces of fruit make an extremely filling and low-calorie lunch. They're easy to take to work and can also be readily found in most restaurants, even the fast-food chains.

2. I have a wonderfully filling dinner suggestion for you. I call it Judy's Gruel. One serving of this and you'll be full for the night. Mash one cup of couscous

(recipe follows) with a baked or micro-waved potato. Eat without any spices, or sprinkle on some herbs.

IMPORTANT—be sure to drink one or two glasses of water with your gruel. Couscous is a grain that can absorb an enormous amount of liquid. Eat it with water and it accomplishes what that high-priced balloon operation does: it completely fills your stomach and makes you feel full.

118

Couscous can be bought for pennies in any health food store, and it's the easiest thing in the world to prepare. Simply boil one cup of water and pour it over one cup of couscous in a bowl. Cover and let stand for ten minutes. Uncover and fluff up the couscous with the tines of a fork. And that's it.

Couscous is an absolutely delicious grain which tastes much like pasta. Indeed, it is excellent as a pasta alternative, served with tomato sauce, etc. I think you'll love it.

3. Water is also useful as a means of feeling full. Always put out a glass of water when you're eating, even if you end up not drinking it. If you are bingeing (eating anything off your diet), I recommend that you drink a glass of water after each item in order to fill yourself up faster and diminish the amount of damage. Moreover, sometimes we find ourselves eating when what is really propelling us is thirst.

4. When bingeing because you're "hungry," wait fifteen minutes between each item you eat. Tell yourself you'll let yourself eat whatever you want, as long as you follow this rule. Not only does this usually succeed in cutting down on quantities, it also gives you a feeling of some control. You may still end up putting on some weight, but you won't feel as bad about it—and that counts for something, too.

On Eating Because It Tastes Good

119

To eat because of taste is to give in to a compulsion, to take momentary pleasure, though it results in long-term pain. On the surface, compulsions appear to be self-indulgent. You give in to the desire for pleasure, be it from alcohol, drugs or food. But is it really self-indulgence, or is it, more accurately, self-punishment? The end result, after all, is that you pay an enormous price.

In the course of any diet, there will always be difficult days. As with any other endeavor, however, you become more proficient as you proceed. You'll find that overcoming temptation becomes much easier with the passage of time.

DINING OUT

I don't know why people make such a fuss about dining out while dieting. Nothing could be easier. Oh, maybe it was tough a decade or so ago, but today we live in a very health-and-fitness-conscious age, and no restaurant is going to be surprised or un- prepared to accommodate special orders.

This is true throughout the world. I re- cently spent a week in Montreal and a week in London, eating out every night. No mat- ter what the cuisine in question—Chinese, French, Italian, etc.—I had no problem anywhere. In fact, ordering was so easy I was often sure the waiter must have mis- understood! Yet each time, my order came exactly as I requested—without sauces, spices or salt—and always delicious.

The problem is rarely with the restau- rant—it's with the dieter. Some just darn well don't *want* to diet when in a restau- rant. Others want to, but either don't know how to order or are reluctant to make demands. Let's take each of these objections one by one.

THE DIETER WHO WANTS TO CHEAT, JUST THIS ONCE

122

I know how the argument goes: Who knows if you'll ever eat here again, or have the opportunity to try these foods another time? Besides, everything on the menu sounds so wonderful. And you're right—you *do* have the option of a wonderful taste experience. I'm not saying not to give in to it, only that there's a price to pay. It's unlikely that you'll lose weight that day, and you may jeopardize your diet completely. If you can handle some divergence from the diet without running amok, and if you don't overdo it, an occasional restaurant splurge won't hurt. Only *you* know if you're the type for whom "a little" quickly leads to a lot.

My main recommendation would be to stick to the diet, and to help you do that, don't even glance at the menu. The purpose of a menu is to tempt you to order; that's why each item is so lovingly described. The adman who said, "Sell the sizzle, not the steak," knew what he was talking about. Know in advance what you can have (see section on "How to Order") and ask for that.

If you absolutely must have a high-calorie favorite, ask if you can order a half, or a smaller-size, portion. If not, ask that you be served a half portion anyway, even if it costs the same. And no, don't take the rest home "for the freezer" or "in case company drops by."

THE FRIGHTENED DINER

123

I don't really understand why some people feel intimidated about asking for precisely what they want in a restaurant. Whatever happened to "The customer's always right"? In fact, I have never known a waiter, restaurateur or chef who minded what I ordered, as long as I behaved myself and paid my bill. Restaurants are in business to satisfy customers, and most are extremely gracious about accommodating special needs. You simply have to be determined to get what you want.

And this is where most people run into trouble. Many diners are reluctant to specify anything out of the ordinary. They don't want to cause trouble or make waves; they don't want to draw attention to themselves. I always answer this by saying, "If you had heart disease or diabetes, wouldn't you make sure that whatever dietary restrictions you had to observe were met?" Of course you would, and without hesitation or second thoughts. Well, you *do* have a disease—and a disease that can lead to many others. Don't wait till you develop them to make your requirements known.

HOW TO ORDER

The most important thing to remember is to be very specific about what you want, then check to see that your waiter has understood.

I do the same thing everywhere I go: I leave the menu unopened, and ask the waiter what kind of fresh fish he has that day. I then ask what fresh vegetables are on hand. From that, I make my selection. I order the fish baked, steamed or broiled, with absolutely nothing on it. Whatever vegetables they have in fancy preparations, I order plain. Usually I also have a baked potato (nothing in it or on it—order it unopened) and some salad (plain vegetables, no dressing, no croutons).

You are not asking the restaurant to go to any trouble for you. There is nothing extra for them to do—indeed, there are one or two fewer steps.

Restaurants, even in the smaller towns, have been radically altered by the fitness craze. Diet-conscious diners are changing menus by demanding a greater variety of healthy, low-calorie foods. You will find diet drinks, sugar and salt substitutes, caffeine-free coffee, whole grain breads, fresh fruit and low-cal salad dressings in practically any restaurant you visit.

Here are some additional tips about ordering meals:

1. Though chicken is as acceptable as fish, you are better off ordering fish, which is always prepared to order. Because of its lengthier preparation time, chicken is usually partially prepared earlier in the day. This means marinades, sauces, etc., that you would be wiser to avoid.

2. Always order à la carte. Yes, it's more expensive than table d'hôte, but there's no way you're not going to eat all those courses if they're coming to you. Often you'll end up eating something you don't much like, too, since it came with the meal.

3. Juice, fresh fruit and dry whole wheat toast make a fine breakfast, available anywhere.

Business people are sometimes concerned about making special orders during business lunches, and since meals and deals often go together, they may be facing this problem a lot. My experience has been that no defensiveness is necessary. In today's health-oriented climate, I think a client would be more likely to look askance at excess than at restraint. What's so embarrassing about taking care of yourself? The likelihood is that the other person has a health regimen of his own.

Of course, if at all possible, you'd be wise to avoid restaurants altogether. Yes, I know—you want to live a normal life, and eating out is such a social thing. . . . All this is true; it's fine, it's reasonable—but you want to lose weight. A normal life is appropriate when you're at a normal weight. Until then, eating in restaurants ranges anywhere from temptation to torture. I suggest you make things easier on yourself.

FLYING FAT-FREE

126   There is one other category of dining out that should be discussed, and that's eating on a plane. Again, the solution is easy. Airlines are required by law to offer special meals to those who request them, and as long as you give them at least twenty-four hours' notice, you can order salt-free, low-cholesterol, low-calorie, vegetarian or diabetic meals. I suggest you order none of them, but instead request a fresh fruit plate. All the airlines have them, and usually they are filled with the freshest, most exotic fruit. I've been served kiwis, fresh pineapple, strawberries, etc., in addition to the usual melons, apples, oranges and bananas. Watch out for the rolls and pastry that usually accompany them, however; you'll find the fruit filling enough.

Speaking of fruit, if you are taking a flight on which no meal is served, you'd be wiser to carry your own fruit than to eat airlines' snacks. These are invariably deli sandwiches, Danish pastry or salted nuts, all unacceptable fare. Revolutionary as it may sound, you don't *have* to take whatever the flight attendants come down the aisle offering you!

127

ADJUSTING TO THE
NEW YOU

*S*ome excerpts from my mail...

The letter from the lady who lost a hundred pounds and couldn't get into her safety deposit box. Bank authorities thought an impostor was using her name!

And the woman who wrote she had lost so much weight her husband thought he was having an affair!

And the man who was thrilled because at last he could sit on wicker furniture without fear!

Amusing stories, with happy endings— but does losing weight always result in joy? Is there a downside as well? Is there something to fear?

You sometimes hear people say they're afraid of being thin, afraid of the changes that weight loss can bring. We have happy fantasies, true, but there's also the fear of the unknown. Obviously, the more you lose, the greater the transformation and possible disorientation, but even those who lose a few pounds will find that they are not the same people they were.

130

In truth, weight loss *does* require some adjustments. Not just on your part, but on the part of the other people in your life as well. This should not cause anxiety or fear, however; the changes mean improvements in every way. Still, some are easy, while others can be hard.

I will first discuss the "fun" changes, like buying clothes for the new you. Then I'll take a look at the more serious areas, like the changes you can anticipate in the relationships in your life—changes so potentially threatening they can discourage people from losing weight.

YOU AND CLOTHES

When I first lost weight, I went crazy buying clothes. My closets and shelves and drawers overflowed. With the passage of time, I've become a little less interested, but I still check myself out in every mirror that I pass.

I consider it healthy to be interested in your appearance. When I was fat, I went around looking any old way. I was grateful just to find something that would fit. Convinced it was hopeless, I made no effort to look good.

One of the undeniable joys of weight loss is going shopping for new clothes. You no longer have to dress defensively, buying turtlenecks to hide your double chin or sleeves to hide your upper arms, wearing loose-flowing garments or cover-up coats on hot days.

131

You won't have to pull in your stomach when passing someone you want to impress. Or pull down your sweater when you stand, because it rides up over your rump. Your thighs won't rub together; your shirts and blouses won't pull at the seams. These and other embarrassments won't merit a passing thought. Freedom from self-consciousness will bring very great relief.

You can expect to have to learn some new ways to dress. Most of us have prejudices and preconceptions about what we can and cannot wear. ("What, me? In spaghetti straps? You've got to be kidding!")

But this is a *new* you, a different body, and you're unfamiliar with its look. You should experiment with styles you never thought you could wear—belts, shorts and halters, sleeveless clothes and miniskirts. I'll bet you'll be surprised at the fashions you can wear.

And expect compliments and attention, which will make you feel great. Learn to say a plain "Thank you"—never put yourself down. You've earned it, you deserve it—now enjoy your reward.

YOU AND FOOD

The greatest thing about eating properly is that over time (yes, it takes time), your feelings about food will change. It will stop being so important to you; it will become less of an issue in your life.

I am not saying that your craving for food ever goes away. It remains, sometimes even as intense, but it surfaces less frequently and does less damage when it occurs. In my fat days, I had maybe three or four good diet days each month, and the remaining twenty-seven were the pits. I have now reversed that ratio: I have three or four bad days a month, and the rest of the time I select wisely and eat well. The problem remains, but the degree of control over it improves.

Because of your history with weight and diet, it is likely that you will never overeat without anxiety, as if each binge foretells your future and predicts you won't keep off the weight. As time goes by, however, each time you stray will become less fraught with significance and you will no longer see it as a portent of doom. It's crucial to learn that you can fall off and GET RIGHT BACK ON, because as long as you can do this, you will never have a problem with weight. A binge will be seen as, at worst, an unpleasant episode, but you'll learn that it means nothing in terms of long-range success. You may not like it when you binge, but you must accept that you sometimes do. To demand perfection of yourself is dangerous, because it guarantees that you will fail.

As for your tendency to blame yourself when you overeat, you really should try to shelve it. It not only serves no purpose but it's counterproductive as well. Accept the intermittent cheat with resignation. Learn to live peaceably with your food problem instead of getting caught up in its vise.

133

Contrary to common belief, a diet is not one thing that you're either on or off. It is made up of hundreds of different behaviors; to gain control of your weight is to make progress along multiple lines. You may never eliminate the problem completely, but you can expect to improve all the time. Keep working at it, and you will see changes—and they will come automatically, on their own.

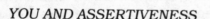

YOU AND ASSERTIVENESS

Being overweight is a form of withdrawal—you withdraw into surplus flesh. Losing weight, therefore, means exposure, and for many, this is fraught with fear.

Weight loss is usually perceived as an external alteration; however, it inevitably involves internal changes as well. When we lose weight, we become someone worthy of our own respect, someone who has undertaken and completed a difficult task. This leads to greater self-confidence and a revised perception of self.

When you think highly of yourself, you expect respect and good treatment from others, and this can be very different from your usual self-effacing, nurturing-others self. Many—particularly women—are afraid of becoming a bitch if they lose weight, as if becoming assertive should be equated with being a bitch. The two are completely unrelated. Being assertive means learning how to get your own legitimate needs met, refusing to settle for poor or indifferent treatment from others. It is a healthy step to take, and usually results in improved relationships across the board.

134

Learning to get your diet needs met can be excellent assertiveness training. It involves dealing with waiters, hostesses, family members, and it contributes greatly to personal growth.

Don't worry about becoming self-centered and nasty to others. In fact, my observation has been that losing weight makes people much nicer. When you're happy, it's much easier to be gentle, tolerant and kind.

YOU AND YOUR PRESENT RELATIONSHIPS

What changes will losing weight make in the central relationships in your life?

There is, of course, no easy answer, no general outcome that applies to all. In my four years in Durham, I saw friendships falter and friendships form, I saw broken engagements and newfound love, I saw some marriages get more intimate and I saw other marriages fail. But I never saw a change that wasn't for the better, no matter how the chips fell.

Overall, I would say that if you have a good, supportive relationship to begin with, losing weight will make it even better. If, on the other hand, the relationship is poor, it can get better—or it can get worse.

135

Losing weight may lead to the decision to abandon a central relationship, to strike out on your own, looking for something better in life. This is undeniably difficult, but it is not a negative step. In most cases, destructive relationships *should* be abandoned if they cannot be improved.

Walking away from excess weight is one form of walking away from misery, and it is frequently accompanied by other forms of leaving unhappiness behind. People lose weight and change jobs. They move from depressing apartments to bright new premises. And yes, they sometimes leave their mates.

The mere thought of these potential changes can be so frightening that many never begin a diet, rather than have to deal with the possible consequences. But it is important to remember that the thin self who will be considering these changes is not the same person who started the diet weeks or months before. This thin person, this new you, will have a vastly different perspective on life. You'll be operating from a position of strength, rather than from fear and feelings of dependence. You'll have a new optimism, a new self-perception, the conviction that life can be good—even when the future's unknown.

My advice is to try not to think about possible problems. Wait till the new you emerges, then let that powerful new person decide.

136

YOU AND DATING

What about those who start on diets while unattached? Can they expect it to be easier to find someone they can love? Of course that's so! Like it or not, fat is not coveted in our society, especially not when one is looking for a mate. With the exception of "chubby-chasers," most people do not want an overweight date. The overweight are considered unappealing and, sadly, an embarrassment to be seen with.

Of course, dealing with the opposite sex introduces a whole new set of problems, especially for those who have long insulated themselves from it with weight. Being attractive may have been what we wanted, but it is certainly not without stress. I consider it no accident that many young women start putting on weight when they reach the adolescent years. Twelve or thirteen is probably the most common age at which women gain.

The night before I left Montreal for Durham, I assessed what fat had meant in my life, and it was clear to me that the only price I had ever paid had been with men. My weight had never kept me from having friends or from being successful at work. But it sure had cut down on my social and sexual life.

I determined that night that if I found myself having problems with dating after I lost weight, I would simply remove myself from the fray. If necessary, I would stop dating entirely rather than having to gain weight as a means of avoidance.

Sure enough, when I first lost weight, I had my share of dating problems. In many ways I was like a thirteen-year-old, learning about men for the very first time. I made my mistakes, but I learned from them— and a heck of a lot faster than had I really been thirteen. On the whole, the learning was even fun. Now men are a happy and important part of my life.

SOME FINAL COMMENTS

I wanted to give myself the very best life possible, and I knew that wasn't fat.

Being thin is unfamiliar, and it represents a certain risk. But what exactly are you risking? Hey, you can always put the weight back on!

Don't look upon the unknown as fearful. Regard it as an adventure instead.

When you move away from something, you must move *toward* something else. It takes the same energy and effort to build a new life as you were previously devoting to food.

138

You must be prepared for false starts and disappointments, mixed in with the excitement and fun. You'll have a lot to learn; you're bound to make mistakes. But you *will* learn, you will change, you will grow and become. You will be who you were meant to be—the best possible you.

PLASTIC SURGERY

There are many excellent books on the market on the subject of plastic surgery, so you don't need me for that. Instead, I will tell you my personal experience with plastic surgery—what it's done for me, and what I think you'll want to know from the patient's point of view.

First of all, my credentials: I've had almost everything done. When people ask me what operations I've had, I answer that it would be quicker to ask me what I *haven't* had done—namely my wrists and my ankles, and that's about it.

I've had my face done, including my forehead. I've had my breasts done—first lifted, then implants. I've had my thighs and stomach done, as well as my buttocks. Even my knees and upper arms have been tucked. You might expect me to look like a patchwork quilt, but instead I look terrific. Everything is firm, tight, up and out, and

I'm just crazy about my body, both in and out of clothes.

OVERCOMING RESERVATIONS

You may have reservations about considering such "frivolous" work. I certainly did. After I lost weight, I knew there was some slack skin, but I had no intention of doing anything about it. It wasn't all that bad, you couldn't see it in clothes and it certainly didn't bother *me*.

140

Then I went to visit a friend who lives in L.A. and whose husband is in the movie business. We were trying on clothes one day, and when she saw my body naked, she blurted, "Judy, you've got to get your body done. You've done half the work by losing weight; now do the other half."

To tell you the truth, I was outraged. Here I had lost 140 pounds, but was that good enough? No! It appeared I now had to lie down on an operating table and have myself cut, trimmed and made to measure —for what? For whom?

"You and your superficial Hollywood values!" I shouted at her, and slammed into my room, where I sat and stewed over the episode. I was getting angrier and angrier —until suddenly I saw it quite differently. I realized that there were no rights and wrongs to this issue; it was simply a matter of attitude. I could take the attitude that I had already done enough, or I could say, "Hey, I'm lucky to be living at a time when the technology for this exists, and I'm doubly lucky that I am able to afford it." Ultimately, it was the second point of view I decided to take, and I consider this one of the best decisions of my life.

Plastic surgery can be viewed as self-rejection or as self-enhancement. How *you* view it is simply a matter of choice.

In all other areas, we feel comfortable taking advantage of advances in science and medicine. Why not with plastic surgery, as well? Your appearance has an enormous impact on how you both see and present yourself. Those most obsessed with their appearance are those who *don't* feel good about it, not those who do.

141

CHOOSING A SURGEON

I started out thinking that I had to find the "best" doctor in the country to work on my precious body. The costliest, the one with the longest waiting list, the one who did the Hollywood stars. Superstars do exist, but I quickly learned that local surgeons can be every bit as good as the famous names, and cheaper, too. Moreover, even the celebrity surgeons can make mistakes.

Obviously, doctor selection is important, and in my opinion, your best bet is to choose someone whose work you have actually seen and admired. Plastic surgery is no longer a hush-hush procedure, and many people openly discuss the work they've had done. If a surgeon did a good job on a friend, he's likely to do well by you, too.

(Please note that doctors usually have specialties, and someone who does wonderful faces may not have much experience doing tummy-tucks. Look for a doctor with expertise on the particular body part you want done.)

142

If you have no access to word-of-mouth referrals, there are several professional corporations that can help. Write or call any of the following for the names of doctors in your area who have advanced training in plastic surgery:

American Academy of Facial Plastic & Reconstructive Surgery
1101 Vermont Avenue N.W., Suite 404
Washington, D.C. 20005
1-800-332-FACE
(In Canada, 1-800-523–FACE)

American Board of Cosmetic Surgery
15415 Sunset Boulevard
Pacific Palisades, CA 90272

American Society of Plastic & Reconstructive Surgeons
233 North Michigan Avenue, Suite 1900
Chicago, IL 60601
(312) 856-1834

THE CONSULTATION

An initial consultation should be scheduled several weeks to several months before surgery; the timing usually depends on how booked up your surgeon is.

It is imperative that you be completely honest with your doctor. If you have medical problems or are on any medication, be sure to give him the details. The consultation is the time to get your questions answered. If you have doubts or fears, express them. Ask about risk factors, how much pain you can expect, possible complications, how long you will need to recuperate and if you will need any assistance at home. Ask how he plans to do the work, where the incisions will be, and—*very important*—make sure that he is personally going to do all the work. Look for a doctor who confronts all potential difficulties, not one who makes pie-in-the-sky promises. If it will make you feel more comfortable, see more than one doctor for a consultation.

Most patients expect doctors to show them photos of other patients they have worked on, and your doctor may or may not be willing to do this. If he prefers not to, that does not mean he has something to hide, simply that he feels these photos are confidential. And can you blame him? Would you want him showing around pictures of your "before" to total strangers?

In any case, pictures can be very mis-

143

leading. Lighting and focus can substantially alter the facts. Even with completely accurate pictures, someone else's results have nothing to do with how *you* are going to look. Pictures may show what *can* be achieved, but obviously results will vary with the individual.

One technique you may have heard of is computer imaging. The doctor draws your face on a computer screen and makes changes to the image, showing what he plans to do for you. This can be fun, but it is not really all that helpful, since no doctor can create exactly the same result shown on a computer when working on flesh.

During your consultation, your doctor will discuss with you whether the work you want done should be performed in the hospital or as an outpatient. Today only the most serious operations are done in the hospital, and most doctors have fully outfitted clinics right in their offices. You should have no fear about getting work done as an outpatient. The facilities are excellent, backup staff is on hand and it's less expensive, too.

Some procedures are too high-risk to consider doing as an outpatient. These include breast reduction, tummy-tucks, buttocks and thighs. Others (face, eyes, necks, breast augmentation and arms) lend themselves well to the doctor's office.

COST

Because the range is so great, varying from doctor to doctor, procedure to procedure, it is impossible to cite specific costs. However, as an example, breast reductions and tummy-tucks can run anywhere from $2500 to $5000; a face-lift can go from $3000 to five times that much. A consultation will cost in the neighborhood of $35 to $60.

145

Get a total price from your physician. How much for the surgery, for the preoperative work-up, for the hospital (if applicable), for the anesthesiologist?

Your doctor is going to want you to pay up front, a couple of weeks before the operation. This is standard procedure. There should be no further surgical costs after this payment, since follow-up care is traditionally included in the fee.

Cosmetic surgery is rarely covered by medical insurance, although there are exceptions when the condition is affecting your functioning. Examples of this are breast reductions, tummy-tucks (if you've got an incapacitating overhang) and eyelid surgery (if excess tissue is affecting your vision).

TIMING

I strongly recommend that you get to your goal weight and stay there for six months before having any surgical work done. One reason is that by doing this, your surgeon will be working with the final version of your body, which permits him to do the best possible job. Equally important, for months after weight loss, your body will shift and change, so why not wait to see what Mother Nature does before putting medical science to work?

146

There is also the fact that giving yourself those six months will increase the likelihood that you will keep the weight off. Weight gained after surgery looks most unattractive, since it tends to clump up between incisions.

You can also have problems if you *lose* weight after surgery. Unless you are young, with very 'resilient skin, this newly lost weight can sag, vastly diminishing the effect of the surgery.

Wait till you've finished one job before starting in on the second phase.

EMOTIONAL REACTIONS
(BEFORE SURGERY)

If you're anything like me, you'll be a basket case before you go in for surgery. Yes, you're looking forward excitedly to the outcome, but surgery is still surgery; anything can happen, and sometimes does. It would be one thing if you *had* to have this operation, but to risk your life for something as superficial as your appearance...

I was so frightened before my first operation that I didn't know until the last second if I would actually go through with it. Spending time with friends who themselves had had operations was of enormous help. They've been there; they can help you through the crazies.

I was never nervous again after my first operation, though I did begin to wonder if I wasn't pushing my luck after I had had several things done. But if you're healthy and in the hands of a good surgeon, there is really nothing to fear.

147

EMOTIONAL REACTIONS
(AFTER SURGERY)

Though we all complain that we never lose weight fast enough, the fact is that the gradual loss of weight gives us time to adjust to our changing bodies. Not so with plastic surgery, which changes you radically from one moment to the next. This may be a change we are longing for, but it does not come without some adjustments. You can expect to experience a variety of ambivalent and upsetting feelings.

For one thing, you will likely feel uncertain about the results, no matter how wonderful they are. After all, you still won't look like Raquel Welch, and you'll be looking at stitches, swelling, bruises and scars. Be patient, because the way you look immediately after surgery is far from the final version—which can take several months to emerge.

What makes this period of adjustment even more trying is that you will have too much time on your hands. Having just had surgery, you are recuperating either at home or in the hospital, and this gives you a lot of time to obsess. And obsess you will. After all, there's a radical change in your physical being, a big difference in what you see, feel and sense about your body. Even washing your face (after a face-lift) or taking a bath (after body work) will be unnerving, because your fingers will experience your flesh in a different, unfamiliar way. You don't feel like *you*, and your mind keeps on returning to this.

148

When you alter your body, you can't help but alter your perception of self. You *are* different, and for a time this feels strange. Time does take care of it, however, and before long, you will actually forget your old body. It will remain only as a snapshot in your mind. This new person *is* you, but it takes time to profoundly feel that inside.

It is important to have people who care about you nearby during this time. You are going to want to talk, agonize, get feedback and obsess. It may not be much fun for others, but hey, what are friends for?

SCARRING

Brows usually furrow when people ask about scars. Of course, no one wants to have them.

Sorry, but it's much like wanting to be thin without having to diet: there *is* a price to pay for the body that you want, and with plastic surgery, scars are a part of that price.

This should not discourage you, since scars are not nearly as obvious as you may think. A good surgeon will be able to give you a very fine scar, and time will fade all but the most visible incisions.

149

Some areas of your body will scar more than others, and happily, it is the rarely seen parts that scar the worst. Because of their constant movement, upper arms and thighs seem to scar the most noticeably, while work done on the face and neck hardly shows at all.

The choice, however, isn't between scars and the perfect body. The choice is between scars and flab, and it's a choice that only you can make.

MY VERDICT

I'm sure you've noticed that I'm quite enthusiastic about plastic surgery. And I'm not alone. In 1987, more than half a million Americans (about a third of them men) had some form of plastic surgery, and the numbers are growing all the time.

I had a great deal of work done, and I am thrilled with the results. I think you'll love what it can do for you, too, if you can settle for improvement, and not demand or expect perfection.

LIPOSUCTION

150

Liposuction is a controversial method of body reshaping in which pockets of fat are surgically removed by a vacuumlike device. It removes localized bulges, and has been most successful in the areas below the waist. In a sense, it is a drastic form of spot reducing, since it aims at those areas that do not respond to diet and exercise.

Liposuction was in its infancy when I was getting my plastic surgery done, but I would have been a poor candidate for it anyway. However, I *do* know a number of people who have had it done, and the following information provides the results of their experience.

The Right Candidate

Liposuction is not a treatment for obesity, at least not at this time. It is mostly for the young and relatively thin, preferably people under forty, with taut overlying skin.

The Right Doctor

This one can be tricky, since a doctor does not have to be a plastic surgeon to do this work. In fact, he doesn't have to have taken any courses, or even had any experience. I'm not suggesting that only a plastic surgeon can do the procedure well, but I think you're certainly going to want someone who has had actual hands-on training.

Moreover, you want someone who has not only technical experience but also artistic skill, since your body is actually being reshaped, and an aesthetic sensibility will help.

If you don't have a personal referral, write the American Corporation of Lipo-Suction Surgery, 1455 City Line Avenue, Philadelphia, PA 19151, or call them at (215) 896-6677.

The Outcome—Pro and Con

Liposuction offers you the opportunity to change your genetically determined shape to a cosmetically determined shape. In many ways, you can redesign your body and make it more to your liking. The method is relatively new, but it can no longer be described as an experimental procedure, and there are thousands of patients, in both Europe and America, who are thrilled with the results.

You should, however, be aware of the downside. Known risks include bruising, lumpiness, wavy, irregular skin, dimpling, scarring, numbness and swelling. The pain, bruising and swelling can last for months, and satisfactory results require a time frame of anywhere from six weeks to several months. You will feel stiff and sore after the procedure, and will have to wear a girdle-type garment for two to six weeks.

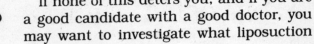

If none of this deters you, and if you are a good candidate with a good doctor, you may want to investigate what liposuction can do for you.

IS THERE A TIME TO GIVE UP ON LOSING WEIGHT?

153

*How to Succeed,
Even Past Forty;
When to Throw in the Towel*

After *The Rice Diet Report* came out, many readers wrote to say that the most inspiring part of my story was that I had lost weight after forty. A lot of them had been under the impression that if you hadn't done it by then, you were probably hopeless.

Some wondered if it was even worth it after that age. They felt that they were losing their looks anyway, so why bother to see a diet through? For many, the prime motivation was to be more attractive to the opposite sex, and since they were past forty, they doubted if they could pull this off, even if thin.

Some said fashions for the over-forty were so abysmal that it hardly paid to work hard to fit into them. Others worried about the elasticity of their skin. The overall feeling was, "If it's not going to make a real difference, why should I bother?"

Is there some point, be it age or circumstances in life, when it is appropriate to throw in the towel? Is this even possible, given the standards of our culture? Can one resign oneself to being overweight?

I was never able to. For me, it just couldn't be—and I hope you have this determination, too. It is not a question of aesthetics—it is settling for never being your best, never realizing your full potential. I didn't want that limitation for me, nor do I want it for you.

Yes, I know you're tired of dieting, but I also know how tired you are of being overweight. You can't bear this endless, draining struggle. Well, the only way you can put it aside once and for all is to get thin.

Mastery over self is a necessity in life, and we see its manifestations continually. We learn not to take something from a store without paying for it, just because we want it. We don't drive our cars at 110 miles an hour because we feel like getting home sooner. We learn from early childhood to adapt ourselves to imperative norms.

In a sense, we can get away with overeating because we don't have to serve time in jail if we don't. However, our day-to-day lives will exact a penance, and in many cases, our lives will be shortened as well. There is a demand for self-mastery here, and we cannot ignore it with impunity. We can eat if we want to, but there *will* be a price to pay.

155

The worst price, unfortunately, is a deterioration in our health, and the older we get, the greater the risk we run. Much of the degeneration looked upon as inevitable is caused by nothing more than poor lifestyle choices.

Those past forty are in the ideal position for SEER—the Sobering Effect of the Elderly Relative. Family members in their sixties, seventies and eighties can quickly educate the middle-aged about how important lifestyle changes are. To see your aunts and uncles bent, sickly and in pain is to look into your own future—unless you decide to change. Walkers and wheelchairs loom ahead if you're not vigilant about how you eat today.

Your body replenishes cells constantly, so it is certainly not too late to make changes after forty—or fifty, or sixty. Forget what harm you may have done to yourself; improvements are still possible, if you start now.

Of course, there's another side to this issue, and that's that many people will not lose weight. They may try, occasionally or often, but they will never do the job.

If you are not going to lose weight, you must learn not to make yourself miserable over it. You *can* be overweight and at peace with yourself—though this requires a lot of self-esteem, which the overweight almost always lack.

156

Indeed, the overweight are usually the first to poke fun at themselves. The overweight man will introduce himself as the "biggest insurance man in Chicago," and women are even more adept at putting themselves down. Humor is used as an unsuccessful defensive measure.

If you're going to remain overweight, this behavior should stop. Don't make jokes about your eating or your weight; maintain your dignity and self-respect. These jokes are embarrassing to others, and they demonstrate a lack of self-esteem. Feel defensive if you must, but don't flaunt your feelings of inadequacy in front of others. It is simply not to your advantage.

Don't let others make fat jokes either, and don't laugh at their jokes if they do. If necessary, look the joker in the eye and say, "That's offensive to me."

Fat people feel they have no right to confront others this way; indeed, they question whether they have any rights at all. After all, they're obviously at fault; they obviously deserve the ridicule. But it hurts; oh, how it hurts.

It's a hardship to the majority that our culture is geared to the beautiful. Who doesn't fall short, even if weight isn't a problem?

Don't regard your weight as a limitation. You can be a valuable person at size 20 or size 5. Why put yourself down because you are the way you are? Again, this is a process. It takes time to adjust to this perspective, because all prior experience and cultural cues work against it.

157

You *can* be overweight and still have a busy, productive life. If you are not going to lose weight, or can't, then don't waste your life in fruitless dieting. I do think you'd be wise, however, to select carefully the foods that you eat. Excessive quantities of healthy food are not nearly as damaging as junk.

The only way I can think of to neutralize this issue is to stop yourself from thinking about it, from buying in. If you decide not to lose (or accept that you're just not able to), stop all thoughts about weight, body and size as soon as they surface. Nip your obsessing in the bud and get on with your life.

This is hard. So hard that I personally believe it's easier to lose weight. I know I could never accept myself fat and just forget about it. Yes, it's unpleasant to have to keep fighting this battle, especially when you have to contend with it for life, even after you're thin. But what are your alternatives? The only alternative to watching your diet is being overweight—and surely that's worse. Like it or not, this is our reality.

My recommendations are as follows, in descending order of desirability:

1. Lose all the weight you need to lose.
2. Stay the weight you are, but start eating healthier foods.
3. Stay as you are and let the issue go. If you simply can't lose weight, don't put your life on hold. Keep busy, look your best and get involved—make the best possible life for yourself, fat or thin.

WHEN HELPING HURTS

An Open Letter to the Parents of an Overweight Child

Dear Parent,

I know how much it saddens you that your child is overweight. This applies equally well to the adolescent as to the "child" in her twenties or thirties. You know that obesity will prevent your child from realizing her fullest potential.

There's also the fact that your children represent you, and an overweight child can be a source of embarrassment. His "abnormal" appearance suggests an emotional problem, since we live in a society that equates excess weight with psychological disorders. You can't help but feel that such an interpretation reflects badly on you.

This issue often leads to ongoing quarrels; lying and deceit become a pattern in the home. The resentment generated on both sides can last for years. To the parent, the child is both a disappointment and a challenge, and most parents feel they cannot leave the issue alone. They are bound and determined to "help" (read "make") their child lose weight.

160

In their quest to effect this change, they leave no stone unturned. They cajole, threaten and bribe; they drag the child to specialists of all sorts. Most often, none of this helps.

Certainly threats and privations do not work. As for incentives, I have nothing against them, except that I have never known them to be effective. My mother offered me as much as a hundred dollars for every pound I lost, but much as I yearned for the money, I couldn't do it.

Moreover, offering incentives ties you in to your child's diet in a way that is not appropriate. If she cheats, not only does she remain overweight, she also lets you down. This only increases the pressure and despair that she feels. You're better off to offer support without any more direct involvement.

I do not fault you, parents, for your very valid concern. Your overweight child *is* at a disadvantage in life. But though well intentioned, your helping can hurt. It hurts your child on an emotional level, and it harms your long-range objectives as well.

If your child has a physiological disorder, by all means seek professional help. And if she wants counseling, do your best to see that she gets it. But apart from that, the best advice I can give you is to butt out. Say *once* that you'll be happy to help in any way you can; then, no matter how much it grieves you, I urge you to let the matter drop. What you see as help, your child perceives as persecution; to her, you're barging into very personal terrain. (It can be particularly hard on an overweight female child to have a slim and chic mother. Have you ever noticed how many of the movie stars have overweight kids?)

161

If anyone is really unhappy about excess weight, it is the person who is carrying it. And ultimately, it must be your child's decision to change. This is not something you can do for her, nor is there anything you can do to make it happen.

I know, it's very hard to sit back and do nothing, but if you're trying everything and accomplishing nothing, you might as well skip the whole thing. It's important to salvage your own peace of mind, even if you cannot help your child.

There is, however, one important difference you can make: keep only healthy foods in the house, and set an example for your child. How can you expect her to limit herself to salads when everyone else at the table is digging into the lasagna? By keeping on hand only the most nutritious of foods, you will help make dieting significantly easier. True, bad foods are available outside, but most of a child's eating is done with the family at home.

You must help your children develop desirable food habits. What you buy, they will eat; what you feed them, they will learn to like.

162

Children form eating habits and preferences well before they enter school, usually by age two or three. Train them to like fruits, grains and vegetables. Give them broiled chicken and fish instead of hot dogs, pork or beef. Tell them blueberries and raisins are a treat, rather than giving unhealthy foods "treat" status. Kids will think that something is a treat simply because you tell them it is. Hey, they believe in Santa Claus!

Of course, age is a factor in all this. The young will accept what they're given and appreciate anything you feed them. Adolescents will already have formed certain eating habits, and changing their ways will be more difficult, but certainly not impossible. Kids care how they look, especially in the teenage years, and it can be very unpleasant for them to be different from the crowd. Moreover, theirs is a generation much more knowledgeable about nutrition than was ours. You may be surprised at the degree of cooperation that you get.

Four out of five overweight children do not grow out of it; for most, childhood chubbiness gets even worse. If you bring up your children to eat properly (all of them, not just those with a weight problem), you will be doing them the greatest favor of their lives.

There's even a promising bonus: recent research indicates that by feeding your child a diet of healthy, natural foods, you can raise his IQ by as much as thirty-five points!

One more suggestion. Why not show your child this chapter, and ask her for her opinion of it. Forget your need to bring about changes; just listen to what she says. This is a very emotionally charged issue, and open discussion may be of some help.

Thanks for listening.

Sincerely,

Judy

163

BITS AND PIECES

This chapter contains all those odds and ends of information that don't seem to fit in anywhere else.

GASTRO-PORN

Ours is a schizophrenic society—one which exhorts us to eat while demanding that we be thin. Billions of dollars are spent annually on urging us to eat; every turn in the road or on the dial exposes us to still another lure. To stick with a diet, you must literally defy your environment.

The food industry doesn't just tap into human appetites, but into human curiosity as well. There are always "new" things on the market or on the menu, in an effort to hold the buyer's interest.

I consider it crucial for you to protect yourself, insofar as possible, from the ubiquitousness of food cues. Avoid anything to do with the topic of food. Your desire for food is partly spontaneous but largely manufactured—and the latter is the part you can control.

Don't read the food sections of your newspaper; don't read restaurant reviews. Don't leaf through cents-off coupons—believe me, you'll end up saving far more.

166

Most important of all, don't talk about food. If others do, change the subject. If you set your drool mechanism aside for a moment and really listen to a conversation about food, you'll discover that food is really a very boring topic. Who cares if something is sautéed or steamed; who cares what's gratinéed over the top?

Talking about food stimulates your appetite, and that's something you can't afford. Why create desires that would harm you to fulfill?

Also, buy your fruits and vegetables in produce stores, instead of supermarkets, where you're exposed to a myriad of foods you can't eat. Don't look at what you're not allowed to eat. Don't pick up boxes to examine a tempting new product. Make things easier on yourself.

ENTERTAINING

I personally never serve anything to a guest that I wouldn't eat myself, which leaves out a lot of foods. My reason has nothing to do with diet, but with health. I don't want my friends and loved ones to eat the foods I know are bad for them—anyway, not in my house, where I have some control.

Nonetheless, I like to entertain, and my friends love what I serve. My favorite way to entertain is to have a salad/sandwich/dessert bar format, with a variety of items laid out buffet-style for guests to choose from.

The salad bar section contains a variety of greens, tomatoes, croutons made from acceptable bread, egg wedges, cooked potato cubes, and oil, vinegar and lemon juice for the dressing.

167

The sandwich bar offers sliced eggs, sliced chicken, fresh salmon and tuna, tomatoes, lettuce, and acceptable breads and rolls. I usually put out some sodium-free mayonnaise, too.

The dessert bar is beautiful. All kinds of fresh fruit, some whole, some cut up. Half a watermelon, scooped out and filled with fresh fruit salad, is great.

WILLPOWER

I detest the word "willpower." What the heck does it mean, anyway? If you're on a perfect diet for six days, then blow it in the seventh, does that mean you have no willpower? Does anything short of perfection mean a fatal flaw?

It seems to me that the term "willpower" serves mostly as self-flagellation ("I just don't have any willpower") or as criticism ("Why can't you show some willpower for a change?"). The heck with that!

The demand for perfection produces anxiety and guilt; if success is defined as flawlessness, it becomes inevitable that you will fail. You are, after all, a person with a food problem. It is your unrealistic expectations that are at fault, not your ability to diet.

168

Forget willpower. All that's required is an ongoing commitment to your goal. Persistence, not perfection, is the trait that will get you thin.

MEALTIME MISCELLANY

1. It is usually recommended that you eat your heaviest meal in the morning so that you can work it off during the day. This is fine if you happen to like a heavy meal in the morning. If it's not your natural pattern, however, you may end up eating a big meal at breakfast—and your usual large meal at night.

   I am among those who prefer the largest meal at dinner, and I can't see that it's hurt me any over the years. I enjoy looking forward to it during the day, and I find it takes the edge off my appetite, usually forestalling any additional eating I may be tempted to do at night.

   This is not an issue where there are rights or wrongs. Like daytime people or night owls, we all seem to have natural rhythms about some biological needs. Don't try to fit yourself into someone else's pattern; find your own.

2. If you absolutely crave something, and you know you're going to end up eating it, then hold off till your next meal and have it then. This is far preferable to between-meal snacking.

3. Try never to eat when you're tense, up-tight or angry. Tension doesn't permit you to enjoy your meal—often you hardly even taste it—and it also prevents your body from assimilating food well.

169

4. Before undertaking any diet, take a look at your history and see what you can reasonably expect from yourself now.

For example, I am occasionally tempted to fast, but historically I have never made it through more than one day, at which point I don't just break the diet, I go berserk. I hate fasting; I look forward to meals, no matter how minimal. It depresses me to go without completely. Yet every so often I'll talk myself into the benefits of fasting, and every single time it ends up the same way. Observe what you can about your own patterns of dieting. Learn from history; don't ignore it.

5. Don't worry if you eat up until the very last second before starting a diet. It doesn't "mean" anything. Most particularly, it doesn't mean that your chances are almost nil. Before going on the Rice

Diet, I ate my way from Montreal to North Carolina, stopping at virtually every fast-food joint along the way. Still, once I began the diet, I took it very seriously. It is important not to let yourself make dire predictions based on nothing at all. There are very few people who *don't* overeat just before starting a diet.

ONE-LINERS

170

1. Be careful whom you take advice from; inevitably those fatter than you will tell you that you look gaunt.
2. Take photos recording your progress— back, front, sides and facial close-ups.
3. Amazingly, many people have only a vague idea of how tall they are; most are off an inch or more. Since your "ideal" weight correlates to your height, this is something you should check out.

SPIRITUAL GUIDANCE
AND PRAYER

I remember clearly the night I knelt beside my bed and passionately asked God to help me lose weight. This was a particularly desperate measure, because I didn't believe in God at the time. I do now, and have ever since I lost weight, which was in many ways a transcendental experience. I quite literally changed bodies, and in doing so, I found God.

Religion is not, as some believe, the purview of the uneducated and the weak. Ninety-six percent of Americans believe in God, and this includes our most admired citizens. According to *Forbes* magazine, 65 percent of the nation's top executives regularly attend church or synagogue, and pollster Louis Harris reports that 40 percent of millionaires rate religion as "very important" to them.

What does this have to do with diet? Absolutely everything, I believe. All religions view the body as the temple of the soul; excess is regarded as an abuse, an affront to God. You need an uncontaminated body for a higher consciousness, and it can be seen as a spiritual obligation to keep your body in a clean and healthy state so that you can help build a better world. It is hard to lose weight for vanity alone; seeing it as cosmically significant can help you do the job.

172

The only real "willpower" is God's will for us, and God does not intend for us to be uncomfortable or unhappy. Eating properly provides physical, mental and spiritual balance.

The Bible offers not only guidance but clear direction about what man was meant to eat. Genesis 1:29 states, "Behold, I have given you every herb-bearing seed which is upon the face of all the earth and every tree in which is the fruit of a tree yielding seed. To you it shall be for meat." After the flood, God permitted us to eat animal flesh as well: "Every swarming creature that lives shall be yours to eat; like grass vegetation, I have given you all."

The religion of the Bible is essentially scientific; its principles are formulas that work, which is why it has endured for millennia. The foods intended for man are those that were found in the Garden of Eden. Pray to achieve such a back-to-basics kind of eating.

I believe that of all the tools available to

the dieter, prayer is the most effective. When we pray, we ask God to intervene in our lives, to take an interest in the things that matter to us. Our eating habits affect our lives and our very essence—it is neither trivial nor frivolous to include this issue in our prayers. We are simply asking God to help us become all that He would have us be. Prayer is a response to the challenges we face in life, and dieting is an important challenge that should not be exempt.

Prayer clarifies what we hope and intend to do; it fortifies our commitment. Ask God for the strength, courage and ability to do what He would have you do. It's easier to say No to passing temptations in the name of a higher Yes.

I believe in being very specific when you pray; verbalize exactly what you want. My usual prayer is for a perfect diet day, and it's a prayer I repeat literally dozens of times a day.

It is especially important to pray in the face of imminent failure—when you're about to eat something you know will do you harm. Even though you're not feeling cooperative at that moment, ask God to help you get past this difficult time. You'll be amazed at how often something intercedes and prevents you from eating.

I also think it is important to cultivate a grateful heart and a thankful mind. There is always so much to be thankful for, if only one remembers to be thankful and puts aside worries and gripes. Whenever you have a spare moment, say the words "Thank You, God," then let your mind drift to the many, many things you have to be grateful for. We renew our strength when we remember our resources, and we are closest to God when we feel happy and satisfied.

174

All too often, we focus on our bodies, overlooking our inner world, yet God is surely our most important resource. Whether you're a believer or not, you've got nothing to lose by trying. After all, in your search to be thin, you've tried virtually everything else, including the dangerous and the radical. Adding prayer to your repertoire surely cannot hurt.

I believe that losing weight, being your best, is a transcendental experience. To eat the way you were meant to eat is to find God, to find the God within you.

I'll admit it flat out, I'm a fanatic. I believe that proper eating can change not only your life, it can change the world. To bring your true self to light is to bring light to the universe. A population of healthy, loving, positive people would obviously approach life in a different way. We would be our best, and we would be able to perceive the best in others. We would be as God intended us to be.

I truly believe that proper eating is one path to the Divine.

CONCLUSION

I wanted to lose weight because I wanted to look pretty, fall in love and get married. I never gave even a passing thought to health. Who does when you're feeling fine? But I have learned what can happen if you don't take care of business, and I want to improve my odds.

There are twenty-six known diseases associated with excess weight, making this not just an individual but a national tragedy. We are the fattest nation on earth, and we must look to the American diet as the cause. Indeed, we look after our cars better than we look after our bodies. The resulting deterioration of our health, not to mention the escalating costs of medical care, should be raising a general alarm.

Destructive eating habits cause disease, but rather than give up our fond indulgences, we tell ourselves that degenerative diseases are inevitable, and that the aging process necessarily means deterioration and pain. This is nonsense. As with anything else, the more you follow the rules, the less likely you are to be faced with unpleasant consequences.

Sure, it's nice to be shapely, but glowing health is even more appealing. I want to stay healthy, be my best, have the very best life possible—and I want the same for you.

Your desire and motivation will be of help to you, but they are not enough to do the job. You must also be willing to make sacrifices. In most areas of our lives, we acknowledge that hard work is necessary to get what we want, but when it comes to dieting, for some reason we insist on easy remedies. We want diets that are "delicious," or "filling," or that permit us to "eat all you want of your favorite foods while losing weight."

It is time to grow up, gentle reader; this is real life we're talking about. Sure, you can be thin—but not without paying the price. There is only one way to lose weight and keep it off, and that is to choose carefully both what and how much you eat. Reasonable amounts of nutritious, low-calorie foods are what is called for. This is a simple cause-and-effect issue, a physiological truth—and the only alternative that works.

Stop choosing wishful thinking over reality. There are no wonder foods, no magic combinations. You will not get thin without serious and ongoing effort. A struggle, for sure, but infinitely preferable to going through life fat.

Put this problem behind you, and get on with your life.

177

INDEX